I0493881

Emergency Water Supply Planning Guide for Hospitals and Health Care Facilities

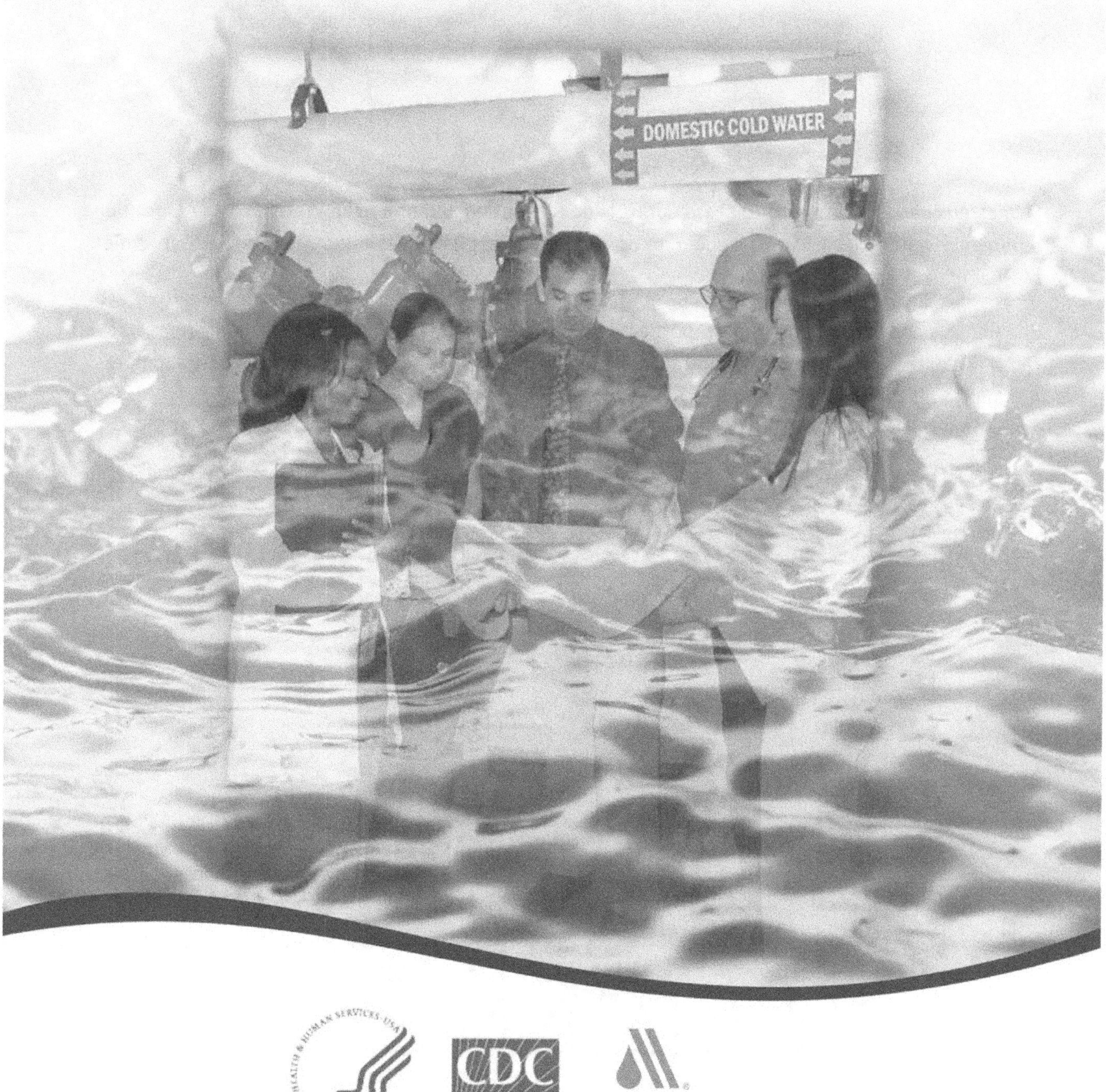

DOMESTIC COLD WATER

DEPARTMENT OF HEALTH & HUMAN SERVICES · USA

CDC
SAFER · HEALTHIER · PEOPLE

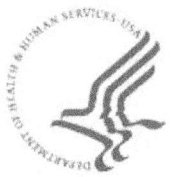

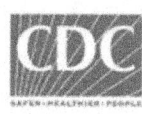

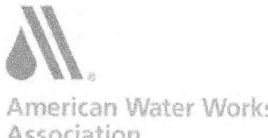

American Water Works Association

220967

Version 2

Suggested citation: Centers for Disease Control and Prevention and American Water Works Association. Emergency water supply planning guide for hospitals and health care facilities. Atlanta: U.S. Department of Health and Human Services; 2012.

The findings and conclusions in this report are those of the author(s) and do not necessarily represent the views of their agencies or organizations. The use of trade names is for identification only and does not imply endorsement by authoring agencies or organizations.

Emergency Water Supply Planning Guide for Hospitals and Health Care Facilities

American Water Works Association and

Centers for Disease Control and Prevention

Acknowledgments

The funding of this handbook was a collaboration between the American Water Works Association's (AWWA's) Water Industry Technical Action Fund and the Centers for Disease Control and Prevention's (CDC's) National Center for Emerging and Zoonotic Infectious Diseases and National Center for Environmental Health.

The following Core Strategy Team assisted in the development of this handbook:

- Matt Arduino (CDC)
- John Collins (American Society for Healthcare Engineering)
- Charlene Denys (U.S. Environmental Protection Agency Region 5)
- David Hiltebrand (AH Environmental Consultants, Inc.)
- Mark Miller (CDC)
- Drew Orsinger (U.S. Department of Homeland Security)
- Alan Roberson (AWWA)
- John C. Watson (CDC)

A workshop was held in Atlanta on November 3-4, 2009, to review the draft handbook. The following attendees provided additional assistance to the Core Strategy Team in the development of this handbook:

- Steve Bieber (Metropolitan Washington Council of Governments)
- Michael Chisholm (Joint Commission)
- David Esterquest (Central DuPage Hospital)
- Karl Feaster (Children's Healthcare of Atlanta)
- Mary Fenderson (Kidney Emergency Response Coalition)
- Dale Froneberger (EPA Region 4)
- Shelli Grapp (Iowa Department of Natural Resources)
- Don Needham (Anne Arundel County, Maryland)
- Patricia Needham (Children's National Medical Center)
- Tom Plouff (EPA Region 4)
- Brian Smith (EPA Region 4)
- John Wilgis (Florida Hospital Association)
- Charles Williams (Georgia Department of Natural Resources)
- Janice Zalen (American Health Care Association)

The Core Strategy Team would also like to thank Zeina Hinedi, Ph.D. (AH Environmental Consultants, Inc.) for her contribution to Section 7, Emergency Water Alternatives, and to Kim Mason (AH Environmental Consultants, Inc.) for her diligent and patient editing and preparation of this document.

Contents

List of Tables

List of Figures

1. Abbreviations and Acronyms

AAMI	American Association for the Advancement of Medical Instrumentation
ANSI/NSF	American National Standards Institute/National Sanitation Foundation
ASHE	American Society for Healthcare Engineering
AWWA	American Water Works Association
CDC	Centers for Disease Control and Prevention
CFR	Code of Federal Regulations
cm	centimeter(s)
CMS	Center for Medicare and Medicaid Services
CT	concentration X time
DHHS	Department of Health and Human Services
DHS	Department of Homeland Security
Dia.	diameter
DNR	Department of Natural Resources
DWTU	drinking water treatment unit
ED	Emergency Department
EOP	emergency operations plan
EPA	U.S. Environmental Protection Agency
EWSP	emergency water supply plan
FAC	free available chlorine
FDA	Food and Drug Administration
FEMA	Federal Emergency Management Agency
Gal.	gallon(s)
gpd	gallons per day
gpf	gallons per flush
gpm	gallons per minute
GWR	Groundwater Rule
HA	health advisory
hazmat	hazardous material
HDLP	high-density linear polyethylene
HDPE	high-density polyethylene
HIV/AIDS	Human Immunodeficiency Virus/Acquired Immune Deficiency Syndrome

HVAC	heating, ventilation, and air conditioning
ICS	Incident Command System
ICU	Intensive Care Unit
Imp Gal.	Imperial gallon(s)
IT	intensity X time
MCL	Maximum Contaminant Level
MCLG	Maximum Contaminant Level Goal
MG	million gallon(s)
MGD	million gallon(s) per day
mg/L	milligrams per liter
MOU	Memorandum of Understanding
MRI	Magnetic Resonance Imaging
MTBE	methyl tertiary butyl ether
NICU	Neonatal Intensive Care Unit
NSF/ANSI	National Sanitation Foundation/American National Standards Institute
NTU	nephelometric turbidity unit(s)
PETE	polyethylene terephthalate
POU/POE	point of use/point of entry
RO	reverse osmosis
TT	treatment technique
US Gal.	U.S. gallon(s)
UV	ultraviolet
µw-sec	micro-watt seconds
VOC	volatile organic chemical

2. Executive Summary

In order to maintain daily operations and patient care services, health care facilities need to develop an Emergency Water Supply Plan (EWSP) to prepare for, respond to, and recover from a total or partial interruption of the facilities' normal water supply. Water supply interruption can be caused by several types of events such as natural disaster, a failure of the community water system, construction damage or even an act of terrorism. Because water supplies can and do fail, it is imperative to understand and address how patient safety, quality of care, and the operations of your facility will be impacted. Below are a few examples of critical water usage in a health care facility that could be impacted by a water outage. Water may not be available for:

- hand washing and hygiene
- drinking at faucets and fountains;
- food preparation;
- flushing toilets and bathing patients;
- laundry and other services provided by central services (e.g., cleaning and sterilization of surgical instruments)
- reprocessing of medical equipment (e.g., endoscopes, surgical instruments, and accessories) after use on a patient;
- patient care (e.g., hemodialysis, hemofiltration, extracorporeal membrane oxygenation, hydrotherapy)
- radiology
- fire suppression sprinkler systems;
- water-cooled medical gas and suction compressors (a safety issue for patients on ventilation);
- heating, ventilation, and air conditioning (HVAC); and
- decontamination/hazmat response.

A health care facility must be able to respond to and recover from a water supply interruption. A robust EWSP can provide a road map for response and recovery by providing the guidance to assess water usage, response capabilities, and water alternatives.

The Emergency Water Supply Planning Guide for Hospitals and Health Care Facilities provides a four step process for the development of an EWSP:

1. Assemble the appropriate EWSP Team and the necessary background documents for your facility;
2. Understand your water usage by performing a water use audit;
3. Analyze your emergency water supply alternatives; and
4. Develop and exercise your EWSP

The EWSP will vary from facility to facility based on site-specific conditions, but will likely include a variety of emergency water supply alternatives evaluated in step #3 above. How the EWSP is developed for a health care facility will depend on the size of the facility. For a small facility, one individual may perform multiple functions, and the process may be relatively simple with a single individual preparing an EWSP of only a few pages. However, for a large regional hospital, multiple parties will need to work together to develop an EWSP. In this case the process and the plan would be more complex.

However, regardless of size, a health care facility must have a robust EWSP to be prepared to ensure patient safety and quality of care while responding to and recovering from a water emergency.

3. Introduction

Health care facilities are a critical component of a community's response and recovery following an emergency event, such as a large natural disaster or localized event such as a fire or explosion. The resiliency of the community depends on health care facilities and other critical infrastructure maintaining their water capabilities during these incidents. To do so, a facility must have an effective EWSP.

The water supply for a health care facility can be interrupted by a number of incidents. In the case of some natural disasters, such as a hurricane or flood, a facility and the water system may have a few days of warning. These events allow more time for preparation which typically speeds up response.

In other cases, such as earthquakes, tornados, or external/internal water contamination, a facility may have little or no prior warning. An earthquake or tornado can destroy critical components at a water treatment plant and interrupt water service for an indeterminate period of time. Similarly, rupture of a large water distribution pipe from accidental damage during construction can result in the sudden reduction or complete loss of a facility's water supply. Because such events occur frequently throughout the United States, the question is not if the water supply will ever be interrupted, but rather when and for how long an outage will occur.

Following are a few actual examples of water supply interruptions at some health care facilities:

- A hospital in Florida lost water service for 5 hours due to a nearby water main break;
- A hospital in Nevada lost water service for 12 hours because of a break in its main supply line;
- A hospital in West Virginia lost service for 12 hours and 30 hours during two separate incidents because of nearby water main breaks;
- A hospital in Mississippi lost service for 18 hours as a result of Hurricane Katrina;
- A hospital in Texas lost water service for 48 hours due to an ice storm that caused a citywide power outage that included the water treatment plant; and
- A nursing home in Florida lost its water service for more than 48 hours as a result of Hurricane Ivan.

Standards of the Joint Commission (formerly the Joint Commission on Accreditation of Healthcare Organizations or JCAHO) require hospitals to address the provision of water as part of the facility's Emergency Operations Plan (EOP). The Center for Medicare and Medicaid Services (CMS) Conditions for Participation/Conditions for Coverage (42 CFR 482.41) also requires that health care facilities make provisions in their preparedness plans for situations in which utility outages (e.g., gas, electric, water) may occur.

The Joint Commission 2009 Emergency Management Standards contain detailed standards, including rationale and elements of performance. Standard EM.02.02.09 states, "As part of its EOP, the hospital prepares for how it will manage utilities during an emergency" (Joint Commission 2009). Two elements of performance for Standard EM.02.02.09 are water-related and address water needed for:

- consumption and essential care activities; and
- equipment and sanitary purposes.

The objective of this Emergency Water Supply Planning Guide for Hospitals and Health Care Facilities is to help health care facilities develop a robust EWSP as part of its overall facility EOP and to meet the published standards set forth by the Joint Commission and the CMS. The guide is intended for use by any health care facility regardless of its size or patient capacity. The four steps of developing an EWSP are shown in Figure 3-1 and are detailed in later sections of the guide.

DEVELOPING AN EMERGENCY WATER SUPPLY PLAN (EWSP)

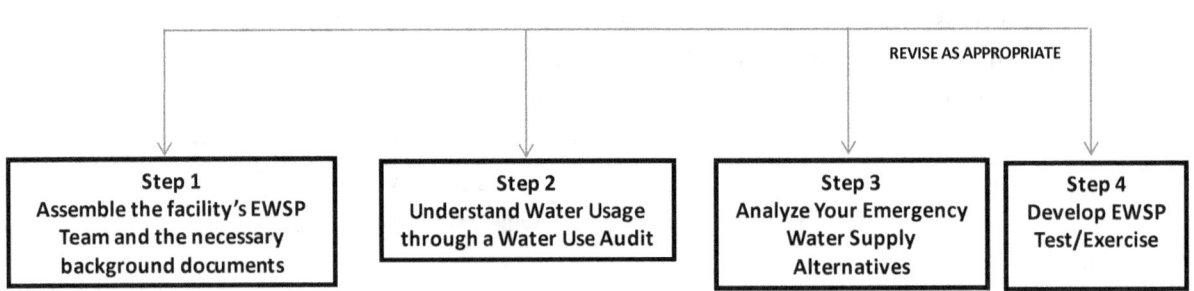

Figure 3-1. Four Steps of Developing an EWSP

The guide provides essential information for developing an EWSP in Sections 4 through 8.

- Section 4 describes the steps of developing an EWSP.
- Section 5 provides a list of key elements for an EWSP.
- Section 6 describes the Water Use Audit.
- Section 7 explains how to evaluate alternatives for emergency water supplies.
- Section 8 provides some important closing remarks.

The Guide also provides information on some advantages and disadvantages of different emergency water supply options. Flow charts are included to assist facility managers both in initial decision-making (e.g., evaluation of how long the outage might last) and in evaluating each of the various response options.

Failure to develop a robust EWSP can leave a facility vulnerable during a disaster. Lack of a functional HVAC system and/or fire suppression sprinkler system could potentially lead to facility evacuation, depending on local circumstances and the event itself. Making the decision to evacuate versus to shelter in place (SIP) is complex and is not an objective of this guide. The Agency for Healthcare Research and Quality (AHRQ) has two guides to help hospitals make the decision of when and how to evacuate a facility during a disaster and then safely return after the event. Information about these guides is provided in Section 9, References.

Appendices A, B, C, D, and E include case studies, an example plan, a loss of water scenario, water use audit forms, and information about use of portable water flow meters, respectively. The two case studies are included in Appendix A illustrate how some facilities have responded to actual water supply interruptions. The project team worked with the American Society for Healthcare Engineering (ASHE) to identify facilities that experienced a recent water supply interruption. The project team then interviewed 12 of these facilities to get information about

- the facility's supply and demands for water,
- the incident that caused the water supply interruption,
- the response process,
- emergency water supply options, and
- the recovery process.

4. Overview of Plan Development Process

The principles and concepts identified in the EWSP plan should be incorporated into the overall facility EOP. It is important that the EWSP and EOP be reviewed, exercised, and revised on a regular basis (e.g., at least annually).

The process of developing an emergency water supply plan (EWSP) for a health care facility will depend on the size of the facility and will require the participation and collaboration of both internal and external stakeholders. For a small facility (e.g., less than 50 beds) where one individual performs multiple functions, the process may be relatively simple, with a single individual coordinating development of the EWSP. However, for a large hospital (e.g., more than 500 beds) where multiple parties will have to work together, the process of developing the EWSP and the overall EOP will likely be more complex.

The following list expands and builds upon the four steps of the EWSP development process shown in Figure 3-1. These steps are to be used as a starting point. They are not exhaustive but are meant to provide guidance to the EWSP development team.

Step 1: Assemble the facility's EWSP Team and the necessary background documents

Begin by identifying appropriate staff members needed for the facility's EWSP Team that will be responsible for the development of the plan; develop a team contact list. Expertise from a range of individuals will ensure a comprehensive and robust plan. External community partners who would play a role in the response should be invited and encouraged to participate in the plan development process.

As noted before, a single individual might coordinate and develop the plan for a small facility, whereas a team including staff from any of the following areas would be necessary for a larger facility:

- Facilities management—this person could likely serve as the EWSP Team leader
  - Engineering or Plumbing Supervisor
- Administration or management
  - Deputy administrator or deputy manager
- Environmental compliance, health, and safety
  - Occupational Safety Director
  - Quality and Safety Officer or Manager
- Infection Control and Prevention
  - Infection Control Director or Specialist
- Risk Management
  - Risk Manager
- Nursing
  - Clinical Patient Care Director
- Medical Services
  - Chief of Surgery

- - o Chief of Medicine
- Emergency Preparedness
  - o Emergency Preparedness Coordinator
- Security
  - o Security Director
- Representatives from External Partners
  - o Local public water department
  - o State drinking water agency
  - o Local and/or county public health department
  - o Local fire department
  - o Water reclamation/purification department

Facilities should check with their corporate safety offices to ensure compliance with corporate procedures.

Assemble facility drawings and schematics. Be aware that these drawings may not be current and water supply piping may not be exactly where the drawings indicate. This emphasizes the need for involvement of experienced facility staff in developing the plan.

Step 2: Understand Water Usage Through a Water Use Audit

Conduct a water use audit as described in Section 6 of this guide. The water use audit will help identify emergency conservation measures that could be used. Also, this audit can identify conservation measures that are easy and simple to implement, resulting in less water use and lower water bills for the facility.

Step 3: Analyze Your Emergency Water Supply Alternatives

Analyze alternative emergency water supplies as described in Section 7 of this guide.

Step 4: Develop and Exercise Your EWSP

Based on analysis of the water use audit and the availability of alternate emergency water supplies, develop a written EWSP for the facility. Practice and exercise the plan. The plan should be reviewed and exercised annually. A "hotwash" and after-action report should be conducted immediately after the exercise. Joint Commission accredited health care facilities are currently required to conduct two general emergency exercises annually. Other facilities may have different requirements. An exercise to include a water supply interruption should be incorporated into at least one of those exercises so that the emergency water supply plan is appropriately tested.

Revise the plan after each exercise if appropriate. Other reasons to consider revising the emergency water supply plan can include a significant facility expansion or modification or the experience gained from a response to an actual water supply interruption.

5. Plan Elements

The EWSP should include the elements listed below. This list is not exhaustive, so other items may need to be considered.

- Facility description—type and location of facility, type of population(s) served (e.g., urban, suburban, rural, mixed, age groups), essential services, types of care offered (e.g., medical, surgical, pediatric, obstetrics, emergency room, trauma center, burn center, intensive care units, dialysis), size of facility (e.g., square footage), number and distribution of beds (e.g., critical/intensive care, surgical, pediatric, obstetrical)

- Water supply—clear descriptions of facility's water source(s)/supplier(s) (including utility and other source/supplier contact information) and supply main(s) and corresponding meter(s) for water entering the facility

- Water demand—both during normal usage, as well as during potential reduced usage during an emergency. This guide provides detailed information about how to understand water usage patterns by means of a water use audit.

- Facility drawing(s)—drawings, diagrams, and/or photos showing all water mains, valves, and meters for the facility. These drawings, diagrams, and/or photos should accurately show main lines for all utilities (e.g., water, sewer, gas, electric, cable television, telephone) and their physical relationship to each other. For larger facilities, a table with valve tags (showing the numbers for each valve) should be included.

- Equipment and materials list—all equipment, processes, and materials (e.g., HVAC, food preparation, laundry, hemodialysis, laboratory equipment, water-cooled compressors) that use water, including location of all plumbing fixtures

- Backflow prevention plan— to prevent possible reversal of water flow and resultant water contamination that can occur from unwanted pressure changes

- Maintenance plan, including valve exercising (i.e., testing the operation of water valves)— Valve exercising is a routine scheduled maintenance program that involves opening and closing water valves to ensure proper operation.

- Copies of all contracts and other agreements related to supplying emergency water and providing any equipment or other supplies that would be used to produce/supply an emergency water supply (e.g., bottled water, tankers, mutual aid agreements, portable water treatment units).

- Menu of emergency water supply alternatives identified as a result of the analysis of the alternatives discussed in Section 7.

- Operational guidelines and protocols that address treatment processes and water quality testing (if treatment and/or disinfection of water is included as part of the EWSP).

- Implementation timeline during an emergency—the EWSP should be part of, and implemented in conjunction with, the facility's overall EOP and Incident Command System activation. The communications plan should be part of this timeline.

- Recovery plan—addresses how the facility will return to normal operations, including cleaning and/or decontamination of any HVAC equipment, internal plumbing, and medical and laboratory equipment.
- Post-incident surveillance plan—guidance and protocol for detecting any increase in health care-associated illness due to biological and/or chemical agents in the water.
- EWSP evaluation and improvement strategy—guidance and protocols for testing and exercising the plan and refining it (e.g., use of after-action reports).

6. Water Use Audit

The Water Use Audit provides a series of steps/actions that will enable a facility to determine its critical emergency water needs by quantifying the details of its water use and determining where it is essential and where it can be restricted. This audit also can be beneficial by helping identify water conservation measures in day-to-day operations. Reducing routine water usage can conserve energy, reduce long-term costs, and increase a facility's resiliency during an emergency.

6.1. Water Use Audit Work Plan

As part of the development of an emergency response plan, the facility needs to

- Develop working estimates of the quantity and quality of the water requirements of its various facility functions.
- Identify which functions are essential to protect patients' health and safety and should remain in operation. This could include such functions as medical gas and suction for ventilator patients if compressors are water cooled. Identify functions that can be temporarily restricted or eliminated (e.g., elective surgery, routine outpatient clinic visits) in the event of an interruption in the facility's water supply, then determine the steps required to restrict or eliminate these functions temporarily. For example, one step might be to triage or transfer new acute patients to unaffected facilities, although initial stabilization in the emergency department may be necessary before such triage or transfer.
- Develop working estimates of the quantity and quality of water required to continue operation of essential functions and to meet the emergency demands.
- Identify available alternative water supplies, including quantity and quality available; how the water will be provided; how, if necessary, it will be treated and/or tested for safety; how it will be distributed; what conditions may exist or occur to limit or prevent its availability; and how these conditions will be addressed.

6.2. Approach

This guide describes the water use audit process, including how to analyze the data obtained.

A water use audit generally will include five steps:

1. Determine water usage under normal operating conditions for the various functions, services, and departments within the facility;
2. Identify essential functions and minimum water needs;
3. Identify emergency water conservation measures;
4. Identify alternative water supplies; and
5. Develop an emergency water restriction plan.

Sections 6.3 through 6.7 explain each step of the water use audit process.

6.3. Step 1: Determine Water Usage under Normal Operating Conditions

Before starting to document actual water usage, the person(s) leading this effort should

- Identify personnel who will be involved in these efforts, such as department heads and engineering staff (see list in Section 4, Step 1);
- Establish and confirm the points of contact within each department;
- Collect needed documents, including facility drawings, water meter records, prior water surveys, water and sewer bills, and operating records of water-using equipment. Assemble the facility's water use records, including water bills from at least the past 12 months in order to get an idea of seasonal variation (if any) in the facility's water use.
- Obtain information about the facility's current and potential future operational needs, under average and surge conditions, as they relate to patient and staff needs;
- Gather lists of all the facility's water-using buildings, locations, equipment, and systems.

The next task is to estimate and tabulate the overall amount of water used per day, under normal operating conditions, in the entire facility, as well as in each individual functional area/department. The information collected should include water meter records for permanently installed flow meters as well as water consumption estimates for each functional area/department based both on usage estimates and on knowledge of actual direct water usage.

Appendix D contains examples of water use audit forms that can be used to assist in obtaining water usage information for various functional areas/departments. Although each facility has unique attributes, a typical facility generally will need to develop, at a minimum, estimates of water usage for the functions outlined in Table 6.3-1.

Where water usage cannot be measured directly, it can be estimated based on equipment design information, frequency and duration of use, interviews with the staff, and standard accepted water consumption values for common uses. Some facilities may be able to use wastewater discharge reports as a mechanism to back-calculate water usage in some areas of the facility. However, it should be noted that in many places, the sewer bills are based on winter water use and may not accurately reflect water use at other times of the year.

After tabulating known and estimated water usage for each part of the facility, the next task is to compare the sum of these tabulations with the actual meter records. Because each part of the facility may not be metered, the combined estimates from each building or section should be compared to the total meter readings to confirm accuracy.

Ideally, the total known and estimated amount of water being used by the facility overall should be the same as the sum of the amount being used by its individual functions which, in turn, should equal the amount from the meter readings. Meter readings often show higher water usage than the sum of the observations and estimates from the water use audit. The difference between the two amounts is due to "unaccounted-for water", which can result from water leakage, uncertain estimates, and missed categories of usage. When no obvious reason for the discrepancy can be identified, and it is less than

20% of the meter readings, we recommend proceeding to Section 6.4, Step 2: Identify Essential Functions and Minimum Water Needs.

When reasonable estimates cannot be made based on usage information, or when the unaccounted-for water exceeds 20% of the meter readings, a facility may decide to use a portable flow meter to directly measure the amount of water being used. However, undertaking a water-use study using portable flow meters is a significant effort. The use of portable flow meters usually is limited to locations where water piping enters a building. Using portable flow meters on piping within a building to measure water usage on specific floors or by specific departments can be difficult due to pipes being located in ceilings and behind walls. Appendix E provides information about the use of portable flow meters and examples of locations where their installation and use may be helpful.

Table 6.3-1. Some Typical Water Usage Functions/Services (not all inclusive; functions/services vary depending on the individual facility)

Type of Usage	Function/Service
Facility Usage	Air-conditioning Boilers Dishwashing Laundry Autoclaves Medical equipment Outdoor irrigation systems Fire suppression sprinkler system Vacuum pumps Water system flushing Water-cooled air compressors
Staff and Patient Usage	Drinking fountains Dietary Dialysis services Eye-wash stations Ice machines Laboratory Patient decontamination/hazmat Patient floors Pharmacy Surgery Radiology Toilets, washrooms, showers

6.4. Step 2: Identify Essential Functions and Minimum Water Needs

After a facility has documents and estimates of water usage for its functions/services it must evaluate and categorize those functions/services by determining how essential and critical each is to the safety and well-being of patients and staff and to the facility's ability to provide various levels of service and medical care during a water supply emergency.

The objective of this step is to create a list of functions/services and supporting information that management can use to develop baseline operating assumptions and determine which functions/services can continue to operate during a water supply emergency and which must be restricted or discontinued. These baseline operating assumptions are used to help choose an approach to obtaining water during an emergency (e.g., drilling an emergency well, establishing contracts with bottled water providers, investing in water treatment technology). Note that facility functions and their corresponding water demands can be prioritized so that the plan can accommodate water emergency situations ranging from minimal to total water service loss (e.g., reduced pressure for a limited number of hours, loss of public water supplies following a major disaster).

Table 6.4-1 provides an example of how information can be summarized for management and planning while determining minimum water needs. Functions should be classified in the following ways:

- Is the function essential to total facility operations (i.e., would loss of this function require a complete facility shutdown)? For example, although HVAC functions might not be necessary in all parts of a facility, they likely would be considered an essential function if necessary in patient care areas.
- Is the function essential to specific operations inside of the facility or a particular building (i.e., would loss of this function threaten patient and staff safety)? For example, are normal internal food service operations necessary, or could some patient care services still be provided without them or, alternatively, could contractor food services be used during an emergency? Similarly, are all normal radiology services critical or could some be reduced to a bare minimum without jeopardizing patient safety?

After the facility has listed its functions and evaluated the essential and critical nature of each, it can take the additional step of determining if essential and critical functions can be consolidated into a limited number of buildings and/or limited areas of a building to further reduce emergency water needs.

Caution: Consolidation of functions and shutting off water to individual buildings or areas of a building requires a detailed understanding of the facility's plumbing system, including locating and testing shut-off valves to determine if they work as expected.

In addition, the facility should consider the following:

- Areas and/or functions that may not be available during a water supply outage (e.g., the fire suppression sprinkler system, water-cooled medical air pressure and suction systems);
- Area(s) that can be used as helicopter landing zones if the existing landing zone is on the roof of a building and the fire suppression sprinkler system is inoperative;
- Steps that can be taken to isolate and eliminate use of selected cooling towers and/or to reduce water consumption in critical cooling towers (e.g., increased cycles of concentration);
- Provisions that already exist or need to be constructed to allow for the use of emergency water supplies (e.g., appropriate pipes, valves, connections, and backflow prevention devices to receive and use water from tanker trucks); and

- Steps that need to be taken to allow pressurization of the critical portions of the facility's water distribution system while using an emergency water supply (e.g., closure of urinal flush valves that normally can require a minimum of 30 pounds per square inch [psi] pressure to close).

Table 6.4-1. List of Essential Functions

Functions	Water Needs Under Normal Operating Conditions (gpd)	Critical to Total Facility Operations (Yes or No)	Waterless Alternatives Possible (Yes or No)	Water Needs Under Water Restriction Situation (gpd)	Essential to Specific Operations (Yes or No)
Building					
HVAC					
Fire suppression sprinkler system					
Food service					
Sanitation					
Drinking water					
Laundry					
Laboratory					
Radiology					
Medical care					
Other					
Other					
Total minimum water needs to keep facility open and meet patients' needs					

6.5. Step 3: Identify Emergency Water Conservation Measures

After estimating the normal water usage patterns for its various functions and services, the facility must determine what emergency water conservation measures can be used to reduce or eliminate water usage within each of its departments in order to meet its minimum water needs. The facility then can calculate the total amount of water that can be conserved by implementing specific measures.

Some examples of potential water conservation measures for use when it is appropriate, safe, and possible to do so include:

- Canceling elective procedures;
- Limiting radiology developers to essential use only;

- Using waterless hand hygiene products according to established guidelines;
- Limiting soap-and-water hand washing;
- Sponge-bathing patients;
- Using disposable sterile supplies;
- Using portable toilets (e.g., for staff and/or visitors);
- Transferring noncritical patients to unaffected facilities;
- Limiting the number of Emergency Department (ED) patients and/or using the ED to triage patients for transfer to other appropriate facilities (Note: the need for this will depend on the duration of the water supply interruption);
- Using single-use dialyzers and suspending the hemodialyzer re-use program (for dialysis facilities that usually reprocess hemodialyzers for reuse);
- Postponing physiotherapy services that require hydrotherapy; and
- Shutting off the water supply to buildings that do not support critical functions.

Departments can also consider developing long-range plans to replace equipment dependent upon water (e.g., switching from water-cooled to air- cooled equipment).

6.6. Step 4: Identify Emergency Water Supply Options

After identifying water conservation measures and determining the amount of water that can be conserved, it is necessary to explore and identify reasonable options for alternative water supplies. During a water outage, efforts to restore or maintain all or part of a facility's operations, including heating and cooling, will require an alternative water supply of sufficient quantity and quality, as well as the means to introduce such water into the areas of the facility where it is needed. Although many health care facilities have arrangements to obtain bottled water for use during a water supply interruption, the quantity of bottled water tends to limit its use to personal consumption and some sanitary functions such as hand washing.

A tour of the facility should be conducted to identify potential storage areas for potable water (e.g., tanks, existing swimming pools, new disposable swimming pools). The EWSP Team should check with the water supplier and the regional emergency management agency to arrange for or confirm availability of alternative emergency water supplies sufficient to meet the facility's needs. Arrangements might include isolation of a nearby storage tank for dedicated use by the facility or a possible interconnection with another nearby water supplier for dedicated use by health care facilities during an emergency. Discussions with the public water department and local authorities should address any plans for construction of new water distribution pipes near the health care facility or the addition of piping connections that would enable the health care facility to inter-connect and use other water as a supplemental emergency supply.

The EWSP Team also should identify what provisions exist or would need to be installed (e.g., appropriate connections, valves, backflow prevention devices) to enable receipt and use of emergency water supplies from tanker trucks. This includes identifying the steps that must be taken to allow pressurization of the critical portions of the system using an emergency water supply. For example, some flush valves to urinals must be closed manually because they require a minimum of 30 psi pressure to close automatically.

Section 7 contains additional information about emergency water supply options.

6.7. Step 5: Develop Emergency Water Restriction Plan

After critical functions and water needs, emergency water conservation measures, and emergency water supply options are determined, a written emergency water restriction plan should be developed. Such a plan can help greatly in guiding decision-making and appropriate response actions during a loss of incoming water supply. Faced with a water outage, facility staff must quickly assess the availability of water and determine at what level and for how long it can continue functioning.

The implementation of water restriction measures will depend on multiple factors, including:

- The volume of water available from any alternative on-site or nearby off-site sources (e.g., inter-connected water system, storage tanks, reservoirs, wells, ponds, streams);
- The amount of water that may be available from these alternative sources at the time of the outage;
- The expected duration of the water supply outage; and
- The number and status of patients, staff and others at the facility at the time of the outage.

Implementation of mandatory water restriction measures becomes necessary if the expected water supply loss will be greater than the available volume of emergency water that can be provided.

The water restriction plan should include clear criteria for determining when to enact restriction measures and may include various levels of response based upon the expected duration and severity of the water supply loss.

The following are some examples of water restriction measures that may significantly increase the time during which a facility can continue to remain in service:

- Limiting water use to critical services and suspend nonessential services until normal water service is restored:
  - Accelerate the patient discharge process based on sound clinical judgment
  - Determine clinic services that can be suspended
- Employing supplies, materials, and other measures that limit or do not require water use:
  - Use alcohol-based hand rubs;
  - Sponge bathe patients;
  - Limit food preparation to sandwiches or meals-ready-to-eat (MREs);
  - Use disposable plates, utensils, silverware, and similar items whenever possible;
  - Provide heating and cooling only for essential areas and buildings when possible;
  - Close nonessential areas (such as auditoriums) within essential buildings;
  - Consolidate floors and wings having low patient populations; and

o   Check for leaks and correct plumbing deficiencies, preferably well before a water emergency occurs.

To further reduce demand on the available water supply, consideration should be given to limiting visitors and to encouraging nonessential staff to work from home. Limiting the use of restrooms to those with toilets that use a low water volume (e.g., 1.6 gallons per flush [gpf]) may be an option if closing all restrooms is not feasible.

Facility management should establish standing contracts to ensure the availability of emergency support services, such as portable toilets, instrument sterilization, medical supplies, meal preparation, and potable water delivery via tanker truck or other means during an emergency water outage.

Information from the emergency water restriction plan will be used in the development of the EWSP and EOP.

7. Emergency Water Alternatives

7.1. Overview and Initial Decision Making

When the water supply to a facility is interrupted, management should assess the problem quickly. The response to the interruption will depend greatly on the estimated length of time necessary to return the water service to normal. Experience seems to show that a timeframe of about 8 hours is often the break point between a significant water supply interruption and one that could be handled routinely. However, the 8-hour break point may not be appropriate for all facilities; an interruption of 8 hours or less may be significant for some facilities and situations.

If the facility management is not assured that the problem (e.g., a water main break) can be fixed in 8 hours or less, they should institute the short-term response and prepare to implement their longer term water emergency response if it becomes necessary.

If a water main break is the cause of the water supply interruption, part of the initial assessment will be to determine if the break is on the facility's property or within the distribution system of the water supplier. Determining how long repairs might take is easier for a break on the facility property. However, offsite water main breaks emphasize the need to have good communication channels in place with the water supplier and local regulatory agencies before, during, and after an event.

A water supply interruption can lead to issuance of a boil-water order and the potential contamination of a facility's potable water system and the need to sanitize the system. Sometimes a boil-water order will be issued if water pressure falls below 20 psi for a significant length of time. The order generally will remain in effect until satisfactory microbiological results are obtained and approved by the appropriate authority. Microbiological results typically require a minimum of 24 hours to complete and 2 days of negative results are needed before a boil-water notice can be lifted. Health care facilities should coordinate their response and recovery efforts with the appropriate public health agency and water supplier. Additional filtering and treatment of water entering the facilities piping system can provide additional protection in times of a boil water order.

Figure 7.1-1 illustrates the process for addressing water supply interruptions and options to be considered.

The alternatives in Figure 7.1-1 should be considered for inclusion in the facility's EWSP and EOP for outages anticipated to last 8 hours or less. A water use audit—as described in Section 6—will suggest how to reduce water usage during a water supply emergency. Once water usage has been reduced, the following can be considered as options to help meet the reduced demand:

- Use bottled water for drinking—a normally active person needs at least one-half gallon of water daily just for drinking. Additional considerations:
  - Individual needs vary, depending on age, physical condition, activity level, diet, and climate (e.g., ambient temperature and humidity).

- o Children, nursing mothers, and ill people need more water.
- o Very hot temperatures can double the amount of water needed.
- o A medical emergency might require additional water.
- Use back-up groundwater wells (if available)—If the facility has its own back-up groundwater well, the operation, maintenance, and suitability (e.g., potability, ease of distribution) of that well should be addressed in the EWSP and EOP. Facilities must determine whether and how they must comply with state regulations governing use of such wells. These regulations usually require obtaining a government permit for the well and periodic testing of the well's water quality. In addition, the functioning of the well should be tested regularly (e.g., monthly).
- Use non-potable water for HVAC, if appropriate—Because HVAC equipment typically uses the largest amount of water at a health care facility, the use of non-potable water should be considered. However, an important potential problem associated with using non-potable water is that it could damage the HVAC equipment and result in substantial repair costs. Filtering and treatment of the water may make non-potable supplies usable in some situations.

Other actions to consider during a loss of water supply:

- Label faucets as "NON-POTABLE / DO NOT DRINK" because it cannot be assumed that the water is safe to use even if the residual pressure is sufficient to provide a stream of water from an open faucet. Maintaining an effective operations and maintenance program for cross-connection control will help minimize the potential for contamination of potable water faucets in the event of a loss of pressure.
- Use large containers (e.g., 5- and 10-gallon) of water for food preparation, hand washing, and other specialized needs. However, sufficient storage space for large containers can be a limitation, as can the need to use or replace stored water on a regular basis]. Managing the distribution of water containers (e.g., who is in charge, how many people will it take) should be addressed in the EWSP and EOP.
- Use large containers and buckets for toilet flushing. Trash cans, trash buckets, mop buckets, and similar containers can be used for toilet flushing. The filling and distribution of these containers should be addressed in the EWSP and EOP.

Storage space can be a limitation for the amount of bottled water to be stored. Bottled water also should be rotated on a regular basis (e.g., FEMA recommends rotation every 6 months). Section 7.7 provides information about bottled water storage.

If the anticipated length of an outage is unknown or greater than 8 hours, each of the options in Figure 7.1-1 should be evaluated for potential inclusion in the EWSP and EOP.

Figure 7.1-1

ALTERNATIVE WATER SUPPLIES - OVERVIEW

Consult with water utility and other authorities about the nature of the water outage

Anticipated length of outage

8 hours or less*

- Determine need to limit available water supplies to critical functions only, as evaluated in water use audit

- Use bottled water for drinking

- Use large containers (e.g., 5- &10-gallon) for food prep, hand washing, and other specialized needs

- Use large containers and buckets for toilet flushing

- Use back-up groundwater well(s), if available

- Use non-potable water for HVAC, if appropriate

- Label faucets as NON-POTABLE / DO NOT DRINK

- Consider actions that may be necessary if outage continues longer than 8 hours

Unknown or greater than 8 hours

Continued on next page

*If water pressure falls below 20 pounds per square inch, a boil-water order sometimes will be issued and remain in effect until satisfactory microbiolgical sample results are obtained and approved by the primacy agency. Microbiological results typically require 24 hours to complete.

Figure 7.1-1 (continued)

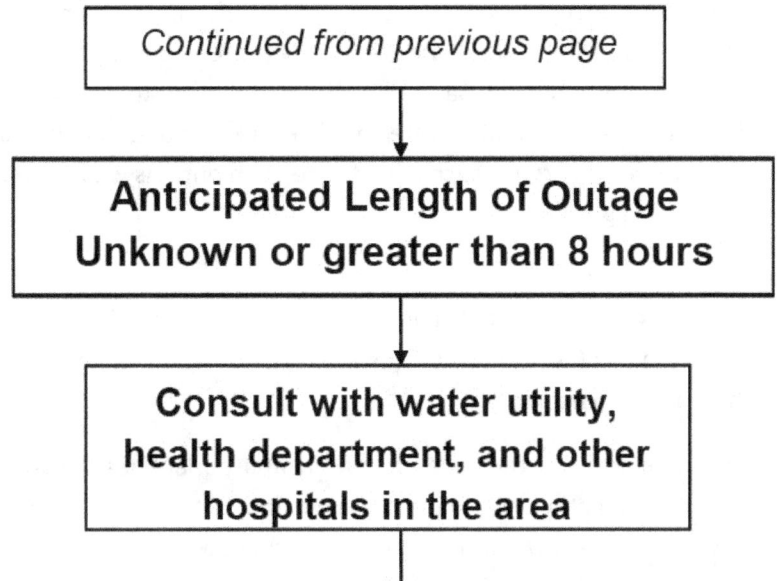

Continued from previous page

Anticipated Length of Outage Unknown or greater than 8 hours

Consult with water utility, health department, and other hospitals in the area

Assess the feasibility of potential actions and alternative water supply options

- Limit available water supplies to critical functions only

- Label faucets as NON-POTABLE / DO NOT DRINK

- Use existing and nearby storage tanks → See Section 7.2 and Figure 7.2-1

- Use other nearby source → See Section 7.3 and Figure 7.3-1

- Use tanker-transported water → See Section 7.4 and Figure 7.4-1

- Use bladders or other storage units → See Section 7.5 and Figure 7.5-1

- Use portable treatment units with nearby source, if appropriate →See Section 7.10 and Figure 7.10-1

7.2. Storage Tanks

7.2.1. Locate Nearby Storage Tanks

During planning for water supply interruptions, facilities should identify and categorize any nearby water storage tanks that could serve as an emergency source of potable water (Figure 7.2-1). Such tanks may be elevated, ground level, or underground and may be located on, adjacent to, or miles from the facility's grounds. Identification of nearby potable water storage tanks requires a visual survey of the facility's grounds and consultation with groups such as water departments, as well as emergency management and drinking water regulatory agencies.

7.2.2. Determine Ownership and Control

Determination of both who owns the storage tank and who controls the use of its water is necessary. For example, a water storage tank on the grounds of a health care facility might be owned and operated by either the facility or the water department.

If a storage tank is owned and operated by the water utility, the appropriate health care and water department staff must determine together whether all, or a portion, of the tank's water can be dedicated for use by the health care facility during an interruption in the normal water supply and if the tank can be isolated to serve only the facility. These decisions may also require consultation with local emergency management agencies in order to prioritize the use of water in the tank while addressing the needs of firefighting and other nearby facilities. All of these issues should be discussed and coordinated with the water supplier and other relevant entities during planning for a water outage.

7.2.3. Determine Safety of Stored Water

The next step is to determine if water stored in the tank is safe to use. Because storage facilities for finished water can have water quality problems including bacterial regrowth and loss of disinfectant residual, it should not be assumed that the water they contain is potable. Excessive water age or other factors, such as entry of dust, dirt, insects, birds, and other animals, can cause water quality problems. Excessive age of stored water can be the result of:

- intentionally keeping the storage tank full;
- hydraulically locking the storage tank water out of the distribution system; or
- short circuiting (i.e., lack of mixing between inlet and outlet) within the storage tank, facility, or reservoir.

Routine water quality monitoring of facility owned and operated storage tanks should be conducted at least monthly to ensure the water is potable in the event of an emergency. Monitoring can include testing for fecal coliforms/*E. coli*, total coliforms, and chlorine residual. The facility should ensure compliance with regulatory requirements as set by the water authority. Storage tanks also should be part of an effective routine flushing program for the facility's water system.

Health care facility staff should be assigned as liaisons to work with the water department staff to establish points of contact and maintain routine communication in order to ensure regular monitoring and maintenance of acceptable water quality in the storage tanks owned and operated by the water department.

7.2.4. Determine What Is Required to Use Stored Water

If stored water is available for use during a water supply interruption, the next step is to determine what is necessary to enable use of this water during an emergency (e.g., pumps, water hauling trucks, hoses). The steps necessary to use the stored water will depend on the type of storage facility -- elevated, ground, or underground -- and its location.

Elevated storage is constructed at sufficient height above the ground to enable water to flow by gravity into the distribution system. No additional pumping is required. If the elevated storage tank is located on the grounds of, or adjacent to, the health care facility, use of the water during an interruption in the facility's normal water service may not require any additional actions unless the facility must limit its operations to critical functions only. In this latter case, the distribution system drawings must be reviewed and a valve isolation plan to shut off the water supply to the noncritical functions must be developed.

If elevated storage is not located nearby, bulk water transport, such as tanker trucks, may be needed to convey the water from the storage tank to the health care facility.

Unless constructed to take advantage of the natural elevation provided by the terrain, ground level and underground storage tanks normally include pumps to deliver water to the distribution system piping. Consequently, a conventional or emergency power supply is necessary to use water from these types of storage tanks. If these storage tanks are not located near the facility, bulk water transport, such as tanker trucks, may be necessary to convey the water to the facility.

If water must be conveyed to the health care facility via bulk transport, planning must include the water hauler and information about sources of equipment and supplies—such as pumps, piping, hoses, hook-ups, and fuel—that are necessary for water use at the facility. The necessary equipment and supplies must be obtained, kept in sanitary condition and ready to handle potable water without introducing contamination, and tested and documented for sanitation safety before use. When bulk water transport is necessary, the existence of adequate parking space, a sufficiently wide right of away remaining free of blockage, and adequate traffic control measures also must be ensured.

7.2.5. Determine the Available Usable Volume of Stored Water

When a nearby potable water storage tank is identified and arrangements are made to use its water during an emergency, the normal and potential tank volume should be determined. This information, together with the water use estimates obtained during the water use audit, can enable the health care facility to calculate how long the storage tank can provide water to the facility's critical areas.

Table 7.2-1 provides an example of Emergency Water Storage and Usage Estimates for a medical facility that owns a 2-million-gallon (MG) ground storage tank. The facility is a 112-acre complex that includes 1 million square feet of medical treatment space supporting a 500-bed hospital, a central energy plant (HVAC), a gymnasium, and other ancillary support buildings. The table provides estimates of the amount of time that water can be supplied to the facility based on various tank filling levels and average summer consumption (in millions of gallons per day [MGD]) under the following scenarios:

- Entire Facility: Normal water use by the entire facility.
- Acute Care (all functions) & HVAC: Water use limited to the acute care facility and to the HVAC units but with no restrictions on use within the acute care facility.
- Acute Care (critical functions) & HVAC: Water use is limited to the critical functions in the acute care facility and to the HVAC units.

Table 7.2-1 illustrates that, depending on the amount of water in the storage tank at the time of the interruption, for normal unrestricted water use by the entire facility, the onsite storage tank could provide water for up to 4.6 days, whereas if water use is permitted only for critical functions in the acute care facility and for HVAC, the same onsite storage tank could provide water for up to 7.2 days.

Table 7.2-1. Example of Emergency Water Storage and Usage Estimates

Area Supplied With Water	Average Summer Consumption	Water available in reservoir (2 MG)	Water available in reservoir (1.68 MG)	Water available in reservoir (1 MG)	Water available in reservoir (0.5 MG)
Entire facility	0.433 MGD	4.6 days	3.9 days	2.3 days	1.2 days
Acute care (all functions) and HVAC	0.422 MGD	4.7 days	4.0 days	2.4 days	1.2 days
Acute care (critical functions) and HVAC	0.278 MGD	7.2 days	6.0 days	3.6 days	1.8 days

Because the acute care facility and the HVAC units account for most of the water used by the entire facility, permitting unrestricted water use by only the acute care facility and HVAC does not provide any meaningful increase in the amount of time the facility could remain in operation. Such an increase could only be achieved by limiting water use in the acute care facility to critical functions only.

To estimate how long a storage tank could satisfy anticipated emergency water needs, health care facilities should perform similar computations based on results from their water use audit and the expected amount of water in the storage tank filled to various levels. It is also necessary to confirm and ensure that only potable water will be permitted in the tank.

Figure 7.2-1

ALTERNATIVE WATER SUPPLIES - STORAGE TANKS

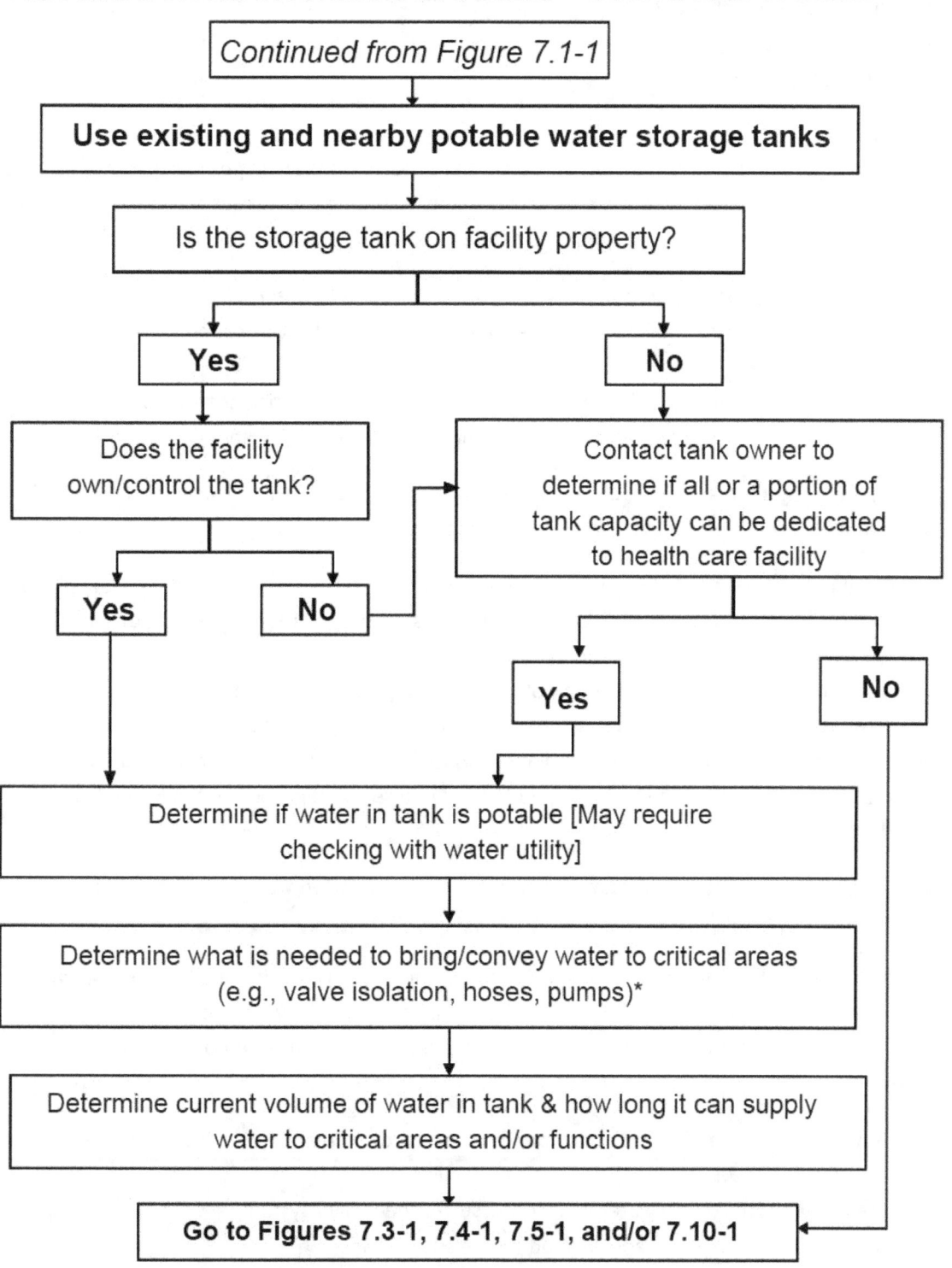

* **Do not use fire trucks for potable water pumping**

7.3. Other Nearby Water Sources

Other alternative water sources that may be available in an emergency generally fall into one of the following categories (Figure 7.3-1):

- Other public water supply,
- Groundwater (i.e., a well), or
- Surface water.

7.3.1. Other Public Water Supply

Another functioning public water supply with sufficient capacity to provide potable water to the health care facility often is the most likely alternative water source during a water supply interruption emergency. To use this alternative supply, the health care facility management must (Figure 7.3-1a):

- Arrange with another public water supply to obtain potable water,
- Determine the amount of potable water that the other public water supply can make available, and
- Determine if the amount of potable water made available is sufficient to supply the entire facility, only the facility's critical areas, or only a portion of the facility's critical areas.

To use any water that is made available, provisions must be made to convey the water to the facility and the appropriate critical areas. These provisions include:

- Closing the connection(s) to the primary water supply (The emergency water supply plan should include diagrams and a written description of all shut-off/isolation valve locations and what special tools may be necessary to operate the valves.)
- Isolating the potable from the non-potable water piping systems (This step should be part of the cross-connection control program of both the water utility and the health care facility.)
- Ensuring that the proper fittings and appropriate hardware are available and can be used to make a connection to the building plumbing or to a selected portion of the facility's water distribution system.

Section 7.4 provides additional information about tanker-transported water if tankers must be used to transport water to the facility.

If the distribution system piping of the nearby water supply is still in service and if there is a water supply line near the facility, the option may exist to make an emergency interconnection with that public water supply to convey water to the health care facility. Use of this option could entail the following:

- Temporary hoses and/or piping to connect the nearby water supply's distribution system piping to the piping at, or nearby, the health care facility
- Use of pumps to convey water and/or pressurize the facility system
- Connection(s) to fire hydrants located on the supply lines

- Closing or opening of appropriate isolation valves to ensure that the water being received by the facility is conveyed to the appropriate critical areas.

7.3.2. Groundwater

A well can provide a dependable emergency source of water for most health care facilities, especially if it has an emergency power supply. Facility management should determine if any wells that could be used for emergency water supplies exist on the facility's grounds or on nearby properties. Such wells may belong to a water utility, industry, or private home and may have been constructed to supply potable water, irrigation water, cooling tower make-up water, or water for recreational purposes or industrial processes. Facility management must determine if the owners of an off-site well will allow its use during an emergency.

If a facility wishes to pursue development of its own emergency water supply well, it should consult with its state drinking water agency to determine if any permit limitations or other special provisions are required. A list of lead agencies for each state can be found on the Environmental Protection Agency website http://www.epa.gov/safewater/dwinfo/index.html and the Association of State Drinking Water Administrators website http://www.asdwa.org/index.cfm?fuseaction=Page.viewPage&pageId=487.

The following are examples of requirements from two different states:

- Under regulations of the Wisconsin Department of Natural Resources, (NR 812.09(4)(a))
  - Emergency wells must follow the codes of the Department of Commerce.
  - All connections must isolate well water from municipal or local water utility sources.
  - Wells for emergency use are limited to wells that produce <70 gpm.
  - Emergency wells can only be used for water supply for ≤60 days during the year.
- Under regulations of the North Carolina Department of Environment and Natural Resources
  - The capacity of an emergency supply well is not restricted.
  - Use of an emergency supply well is restricted to emergencies only.
  - Adequate primary and secondary disinfection must be provided while the well is in use.
  - Emergency supply well piping must be physically disconnected (i.e., shutoff valve) from the facility's water supply piping, when operating under normal conditions (i.e. no water shortage).
  - Emergency supply well piping should be physically connected to the facility's supply piping only during emergency conditions (i.e. water shortage).

If well water is available for use, the planning team must determine if the water is potable or can be made potable, if it will foul equipment used for HVAC or other purposes, and if it is appropriate for other uses within the facility.

Determining if the available groundwater is potable generally will require consultation with the state drinking water primacy agency. If the groundwater is potable, the well capacity should be determined to see if it is sufficient to supply the critical areas of the facility. The groundwater also should be evaluated for its content of iron, manganese, and other dissolved solids which could impact the facility's equipment. If the water capacity is sufficient to supply part or all of the critical areas and if the water quality is acceptable or can be made acceptable for use with the facility's equipment, then provisions must be made to convey the water to the facility and its critical areas. These provisions include:

- Closing the valve(s) connecting the primary water supply (The emergency water supply plan should include diagrams and a written description of all shut-off and isolation valve locations and what special tools may be necessary to operate the valves.)
- Isolating the potable from the non-potable water systems (This step should be part of the cross-connection control programs of both the water utility and the health care facility.)
- Ensuring that the proper fittings and appropriate hardware are available and can be used to make a connection to the building plumbing or to a selected portion of the facility's water distribution system.

A tanker/water hauler may be necessary to transport the water to the facility. See Section 7.4 for additional information on tanker-transported water.

Even if the groundwater is non-potable, it can provide potential benefits to a health care facility in the event of a water supply emergency. These include use in the cooling towers and for toilet flushing. However, care will need to be taken to ensure that:

- The quality of the water does not interfere with operations by clogging, fouling, or corroding equipment; overwhelming chemical processes; or resulting in other damage
- Any equipment or piping being used to transport non-potable water is clearly labeled
- The non-potable groundwater is not introduced into potable water storage containers, vessels, or systems
- The tank or bladder receiving the water at the facility is clearly labeled as "DO NOT DRINK/NON-POTABLE WATER ONLY"
- The non-potable systems at the health care facility are isolated from the potable water systems
- Provisions are made to clean, disinfect, and conduct microbiological analyses on potable lines if they contained non-potable water before they are returned to potable operation.

7.3.3. Surface Water

As indicated in Figure 7.3-1b, there may be other nearby surface water supplies such as a lake, pond, creek, or storm water retention pond that, with appropriate treatment, may also provide an alternative potable or non-potable water supply. Table 7.10-1 provides guidance on determining the treatment that may be required; however providing appropriate treatment is a significant effort.

If appropriate treatment is available to provide potable water from this source, then the available capacity or yield will need to be determined to see if it is sufficient to supply the critical areas. If the capacity is sufficient to supply all of the critical areas, provisions will need to be made to convey that water to the critical areas (as with any alternative water supply). These provisions include:

- Closing the connection or connections to the primary water supply (The emergency plan should include a diagram or written description of where the shut-off or isolation valves are located and what special tools, if any, may be required.)

- Isolating the potable and non-potable systems
- Installing fittings to make a connection to the building plumbing or to a selected portion of the distribution system
- Installing water pumps.

For off-site surface water supplies, it may be necessary to use a tanker to transport the water to the facility. See Section 7.4 for additional information on tanker-transported water.

If the treated surface water is non-potable, there are a number of non-potable water uses at a facility. These include use in the cooling towers and for toilet flushing. Consequently, a non-potable supply can still provide benefits to a facility in the event of a water supply emergency. However, care will need to be taken to ensure that:

- The water is of appropriate quality so as not to interfere with operations by clogging, fouling, corroding, overwhelming chemical processes, or causing other unanticipated results;
- Any equipment or piping being used to transport the non-potable water is clearly labeled "DO NOT DRINK/NON-POTABLE WATER ONLY";
- The non-potable groundwater is not introduced into potable water storage containers, vessels, or systems;
- The tank or bladder receiving the non-potable water at the health care facility is clearly labeled as "DO NOT DRINK/NON-POTABLE WATER ONLY";
- The non-potable systems at the health care facility are isolated from the potable systems; and
- Provisions are made to clean, disinfect, and conduct microbiological analyses on water lines that contained non-potable water before they are returned to potable water operations.

Use of these alternatives will require a significant amount of planning before the onset of a water supply emergency to ensure that the agreements, equipment, and procedures are in place.

Figure 7.3-1
ALTERNATIVE WATER SUPPLIES - NEARBY SOURCES

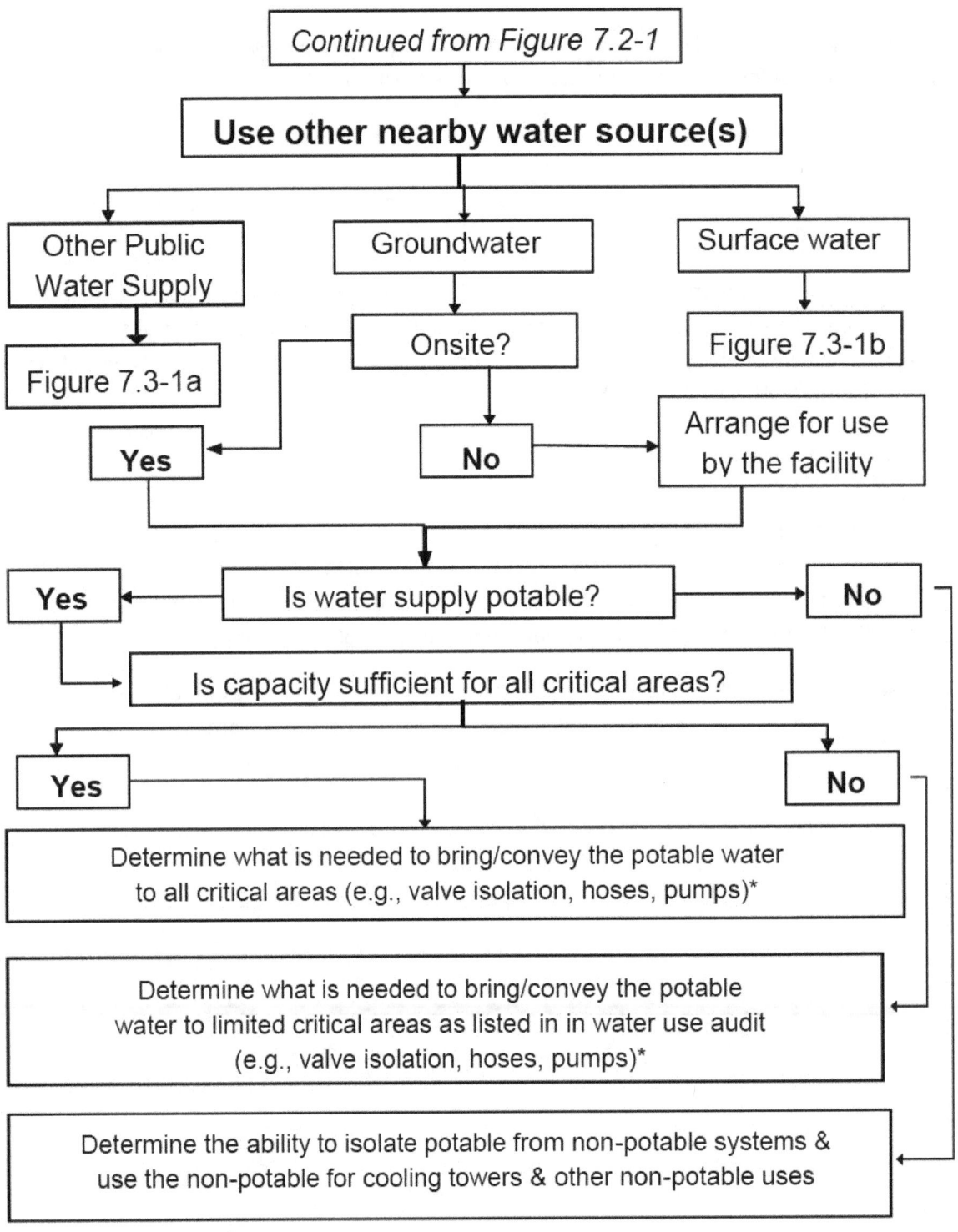

* Do not use fire trucks for potable water pumping

Figure 7.3-1a

ALTERNATIVE WATER SUPPLIES - NEARBY SOURCES
OTHER PUBLIC WATER SUPPLY

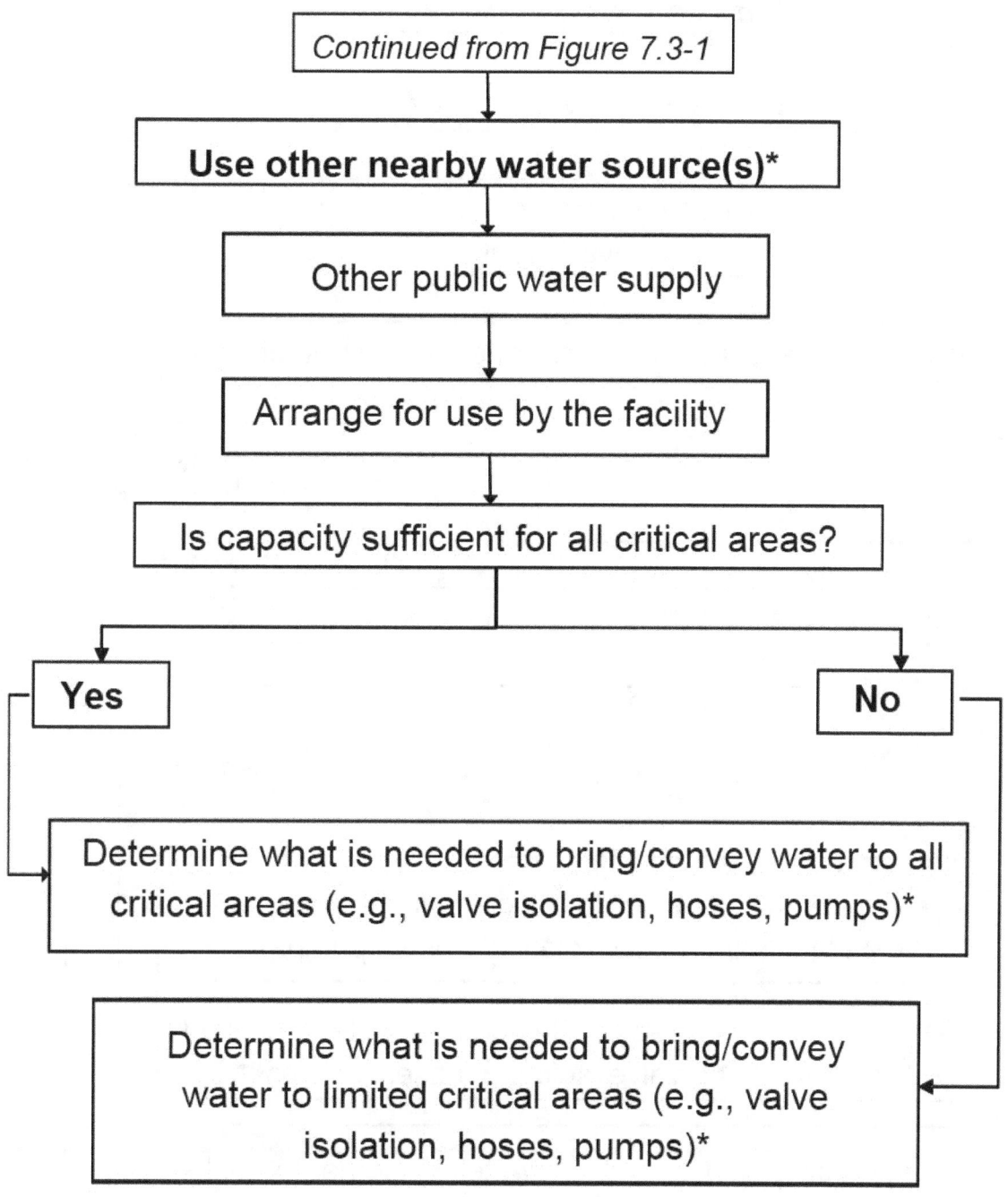

* Do not use fire trucks for potable water pumping

Figure 7.3-1b

ALTERNATIVE WATER SUPPLIES - NEARBY SOURCES
SURFACE WATER

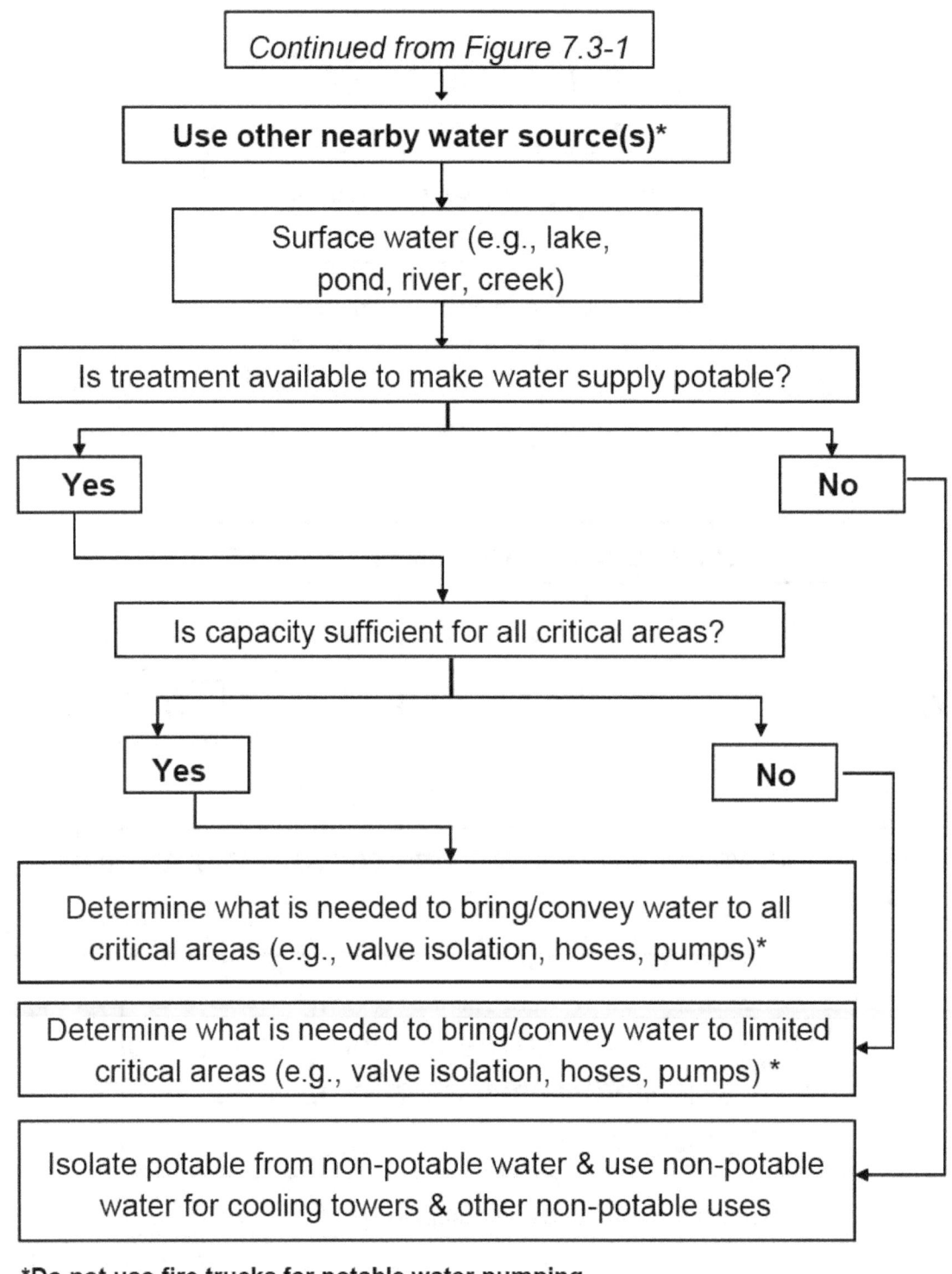

Continued from Figure 7.3-1

Use other nearby water source(s)*

Surface water (e.g., lake, pond, river, creek)

Is treatment available to make water supply potable?

Yes　　　　No

Is capacity sufficient for all critical areas?

Yes　　　　No

Determine what is needed to bring/convey water to all critical areas (e.g., valve isolation, hoses, pumps)*

Determine what is needed to bring/convey water to limited critical areas (e.g., valve isolation, hoses, pumps) *

Isolate potable from non-potable water & use non-potable water for cooling towers & other non-potable uses

*Do not use fire trucks for potable water pumping

7.4. Tanker-transported Water

In a water-supply emergency, facilities may need to rely on a water hauler to transport water to the facility. As indicated in Figure 7.4-1, planning for the use of tanker-transported water involves the following steps:

- Determine if the water source being used to fill the tanker trucks is safe and from an approved source.
- Determine if the tanker being used to transport the water is appropriate for the transport of potable water. The tanker must be food grade certified (i.e., National Sanitation Foundation (NSF)/American National Standards Institute (ANSI) Standard 61), contaminant-free, and watertight.
- Ensure proper cleaning and disinfection of the tanker truck.
- Isolate the building plumbing from the primary water supply.
- Make provisions to convey the water safely from the tanker trucks to the building. All hoses and other handling equipment used in the operation should meet NSF/ANSI Standard 61, be stored off the ground at all times, and be thoroughly flushed and disinfected before use.

7.4.1. Water Source

In general, state drinking water authorities will require that water intended for potable use be obtained from an approved public water supply. This will normally be a nearby public water supply. In these cases, there will be a need to

- Obtain permission for its use from the state drinking water agency, the public water supply that is to be used as the source, and, possibly, the local emergency management agency.
- Identify where the tanker can draw the water from the supply (e.g., fire hydrant, storage tank connection).
- Identify and/or provide for temporary storage of the tanker-transported water.

In some cases, a non-potable water supply source may be used if appropriate testing as determined by the state drinking water agency shows it is safe to use. Testing may include microbiological and possibly chemical and radiological testing.

A number of water uses at a facility do not require the use of potable water. These include use in the cooling towers and for toilet flushing. Consequently, a non-potable supply can still provide benefits to a health care facility in the event of a water supply emergency. However, care will need to be taken to ensure that

- Tanker trucks being used to transport non-potable water are clearly labeled "DO NOT DRINK/NON-POTABLE WATER ONLY";
- Tanker trucks do not contain substances that will harm equipment operations;
- Tanker trucks are not subsequently used to transport potable water unless they are first properly cleaned and disinfected;

- The tank or bladder receiving the water at the medical facility is clearly labeled as non-potable; and
- The non-potable systems at the facility are isolated from the potable systems.

7.4.2. Tankers and Portable Tanks

For potable water, tanks should meet NSF/ANSI Standard 61. Licensed bulk water haulers or food grade tank haulers may offer the best option in emergencies. Smaller portable water tanks meeting NSF/ANSI Standard 61 may be available through local vendors.

Many state drinking water agencies have developed their own requirements or guidelines for transporting water intended for potable use. These are based on recognition that the extra handling involved with transporting water to a facility increases the risk for contamination. In general, these requirements or guidelines include the following:

- Tanks previously used to transport materials such as chemicals and petroleum derivatives cannot be used for hauling potable water.
- Truck containers must be contaminant-free, watertight, and made of food-grade approved material that can be easily cleaned and disinfected. The container must also be capable of being maintained to prevent water contamination.
- The tanker truck transporting potable water must be labeled "DRINKING WATER ONLY".
- Tankers or truck containers need to be filled or emptied using sanitary methods. Preferably, this will include valve-to-valve connections or air gaps.
- Connections and fittings for filling and emptying the tank must be properly protected to prevent any extrinsic contamination.
- Any hoses or piping must be maintained in a sanitary condition.
- A drain and vent must be provided that will allow for complete emptying of the tank for cleaning or repairs.
- Tanks or containers should be completely enclosed and the covers should be sealed or locked to protect the water from tampering.
- The water source should be tested for microbiolgic indicators and chlorine residual before filling the tanker and before discharging the water from the tanker into the health care facility. It is recommended that all testing be documented.

The tank, along with the hoses, pumps, and other equipment, must be cleaned and sanitized. The inside surfaces of the tanks and other equipment should be exposed to a minimum chlorine dose of 50 milligrams per liter (mg/L) for at least 30 minutes. The sanitizer should meet NSF/ANSI Standard 60. The state drinking water agency should be consulted to determine the amount of time that the equipment must be exposed to the chlorine solution. As an alternative, AWWA Standard C652-02 for disinfecting tanks can be used as a reference.

The above chlorine solution can be prepared by adding 1 gallon of 5.25%-6.0% sodium hypochlorite (unscented regular household bleach) into every 1,000 gallons of water. After at least 30 minute of contact time, this solution will need to be drained. Check with the local wastewater utility to determine the appropriate method for disposal of this solution. The tank should be flushed with a safe source of water and drained. Water stored in the tanker truck or potable tank should be maintained at a free chlorine residual between 0.5 mg/L and 2.0 mg/L. Levels above 2.0 mg/L can sometimes create taste issues and make water less palatable. Warm weather conditions can cause chlorine to dissipate from the tanks so more frequent monitoring of chlorine levels may be necessary.

All hoses and other handling equipment used in the operation should meet NSF/ANSI Standard 61, be stored off the ground at all times, and be thoroughly flushed and disinfected before use. Hoses should be capped at each end or connected together when not in use.

7.4.3. Isolation of the Building Plumbing

Before the building plumbing can be pressurized with water from the tanker-truck or other back-up water supply, the connection to the primary water supply should be closed. Note that some health care facilities have more than one service connection to the main water distribution system. The emergency plan should include a diagram or written description of shut-off or isolation valve locations and what special tools, if any, may be required. This procedure should be coordinated with the water utility staff, plumbing officials, health department, and appropriate regulatory agencies.

7.4.4. Conveying the Water to the Building -- Pipes, Fittings, and Pumps

Because the tanker may need to be connected to the building plumbing, it will need to park close to the building where connective piping can enter the system without crossing traffic areas. Knowing the connection locations will allow for placement of the truck and will help with estimating the amount of pipe needed to make a connection.

Facilities should evaluate the need for special pipe fittings—including any required for backflow prevention—that may be necessary to connect to the building, to fire hydrants, or to other pipes within the water distribution system. Consideration should be given to obtaining and storing hard-to-find fittings and other necessary hardware.

Once a tanker is on site, additional equipment will be needed, including a pump for potable water, a pressure bladder tank, a pressure switch, pipes, and fittings in order to connect to the building plumbing. Fittings, pipes, and associated plumbing should meet local and state plumbing codes and be installed by a licensed plumber. If installation is not regulated by a plumbing code, pipes and plumbing should meet NSF/ANSI Standard 61 requirements for drinking water system components.

Pumps must not exert pressure greater than the pressure rating of the piping or pressure bladder, whichever is lower. Pump operation needs to be controlled to prevent surge or water hammer from rupturing piping and attached equipment.

Figure 7.4-1

ALTERNATIVE WATER SUPPLIES – TANKER-TRANSPORTED WATER

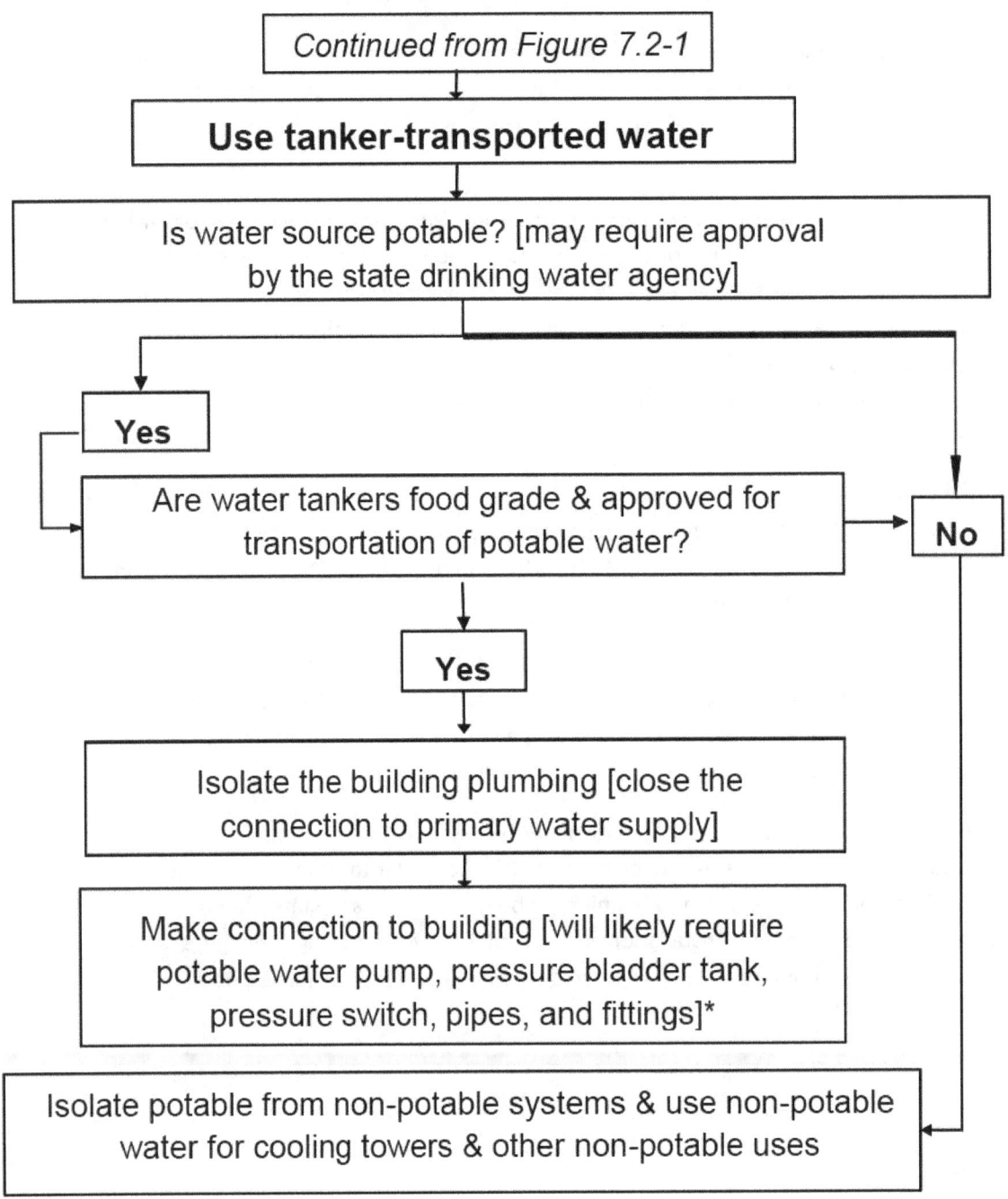

Continued from Figure 7.2-1

Use tanker-transported water

Is water source potable? [may require approval by the state drinking water agency]

Yes

Are water tankers food grade & approved for transportation of potable water?

No

Yes

Isolate the building plumbing [close the connection to primary water supply]

Make connection to building [will likely require potable water pump, pressure bladder tank, pressure switch, pipes, and fittings]*

Isolate potable from non-potable systems & use non-potable water for cooling towers & other non-potable uses

*Do not use fire trucks for potable water pumping

7.5. Large Temporary Storage Tanks (Greater than 55 Gallons)

Facilities should consider acquiring temporary storage for potable and non-potable water for the duration of an emergency (Figure 7.5-1 and 7.5-1a). Information should be obtained about equipment delivery time and set-up, maintenance requirements, and the number of people required for set-up and maintenance. If possible, new tanks should be used because tanks that have contained chemicals can leave harmful residues. Tanks should be cleaned and disinfected before and after use and meet NSF/ANSI Standard 61 for potable water use.

Temporary storage tanks are available through commercial sources and may be ordered and shipped to the facility in the event of an emergency.

7.5.1. Pillow and Bladder Tanks

Pillow and bladder tanks (Figures 7.5-2 and 7.5-3, respectively) can provide temporary storage of water during an emergency. These tanks can be equipped with handles and lifting points which can helpful with positioning. The tanks should have a relief valve to prevent overfilling. Tanks are available in standard sizes from 100- to 50,000-gallon capacity (Table 7.5-1) and can be special ordered in sizes up to 250,000-gallon capacity. Pillow and bladder tanks in a variety of sizes and capacities can be used individually or, if more than 250,000-gallon storage capacity is needed, can be interconnected for a large-scale relief operation or long-term emergency situation.

Because they are collapsible, pillow and bladder storage tanks can be:

- easily stored and transported,
- placed into low-height and space-limited areas, and
- easily installed by unrolling and unfolding.

However, some of their disadvantages include:

- potential depletion of disinfectant residuals during extended water storage,
- accidental or deliberate perforation,
- weakening of tank fabric by age, sunlight, repeated use, or improper storage conditions,
- the need for careful cleaning and storage per manufacturer's instructions after use and before reuse, and
- the need to verify that previous use did not include storage of a hazardous material.

Table 7.5-1. Bladder and Pillow Tank Sizes

Tank Capacity			Tank Pallet Shipping Weight		Tank Pallet Shipping Dimensions	
U.S. Gal.	Imp Gal.	Liters	Pounds	Kilograms	Inches	Centimeters
100	83	379	100	46	36 x 38 x 17	92 x 97 x 43
500	416	1,893	140	64	36 x 38 x 17	92 x 97 x 43
1,000	833	3,785	185	84	36 x 38 x 17	92 x 97 x 43
5,000	4,164	18,927	357	162	48 x 48 x 24	122 x 122 x 61
10,000	8,327	37,854	600	272.15	48 x 48 x 36	122 x 122 x 92

Tank Capacity			Tank Pallet Shipping Weight		Tank Pallet Shipping Dimensions	
U.S. Gal.	Imp Gal.	Liters	Pounds	Kilograms	Inches	Centimeters
20,000	16,654	75,708	850	385.55	48 x 48 x 48	122 x 122 x 122
50,000	41,635	189,270	2,000	907.18	48 x 84 x 40	122 x 213 x 102

7.5.2. Onion Tanks

Onion tanks are self-supporting yet collapsible industrial urethane fabric containers designed for temporary storage of drinking water (Table 7.5-2). When packaged, they can collapse to about 15% of their full size. The urethane fabric meets all requirements for use to contain products for human consumption.

The open-top design allows for easy filling but a cover should be provided to protect the water from outside contamination (Figure 7.5-4). The tanks have two 3-inch input/outlet valves to facilitate filling and removal of water.

Table 7.5-2. Onion Tank Sizes

Part Number	Capacity (U.S. Gallons)	Unfilled Container Weight	Filled Base Diameter	Collar Diameter	Filled Height
Potable Water Tank - 600	600	40 pounds	84 inches	54 inches	38 inches
Potable Water Tank - 1200	1,200	70 pounds	128 inches	82 inches	34 inches
Potable Water Tank - 1800	1,800	75 pounds	154 inches	102 inches	36 inches
Potable Water Tank - 3000	3,000	100 pounds	188 inches	132 inches	38 inches
Potable Water Tank - 3600	3,600	115 pounds	189 inches	144 inches	38 inches
Potable Water Tank - 4800	4,800	150 pounds	224 inches	164 inches	42 inches
Potable Water Tank - 6000	6,000	150 pounds	209 inches	144 inches	60 inches
Potable Water Tank - 10000	10,000	200 pounds	236 inches	144 inches	80 inches
Potable Water Tank - 14400	14,400	250 pounds	260 inches	144 inches	93 inches

7.5.3. Pickup Truck Tanks

ANSI/NSF Standard 61 approved lightweight tanks are available in high-density linear polyethylene (HDLP) (Figure 7.5-5 and Table 7.5-3). These can be mounted on pickup trucks to haul water from a safe source.

Table 7.5-3. Pickup Truck Tank Sizes

Size	Height with Lid	Diameter	Length	Lid
195 gallons	30 inches	61 inches	38 inches	8 inches
295 gallons	30 inches	61 inches	60 inches	8 inches
475 gallons	46 inches	65 inches	65 inches	8 inches

Figure 7.5-1

ALTERNATIVE WATER SUPPLIES - BLADDERS AND OTHER STORAGE

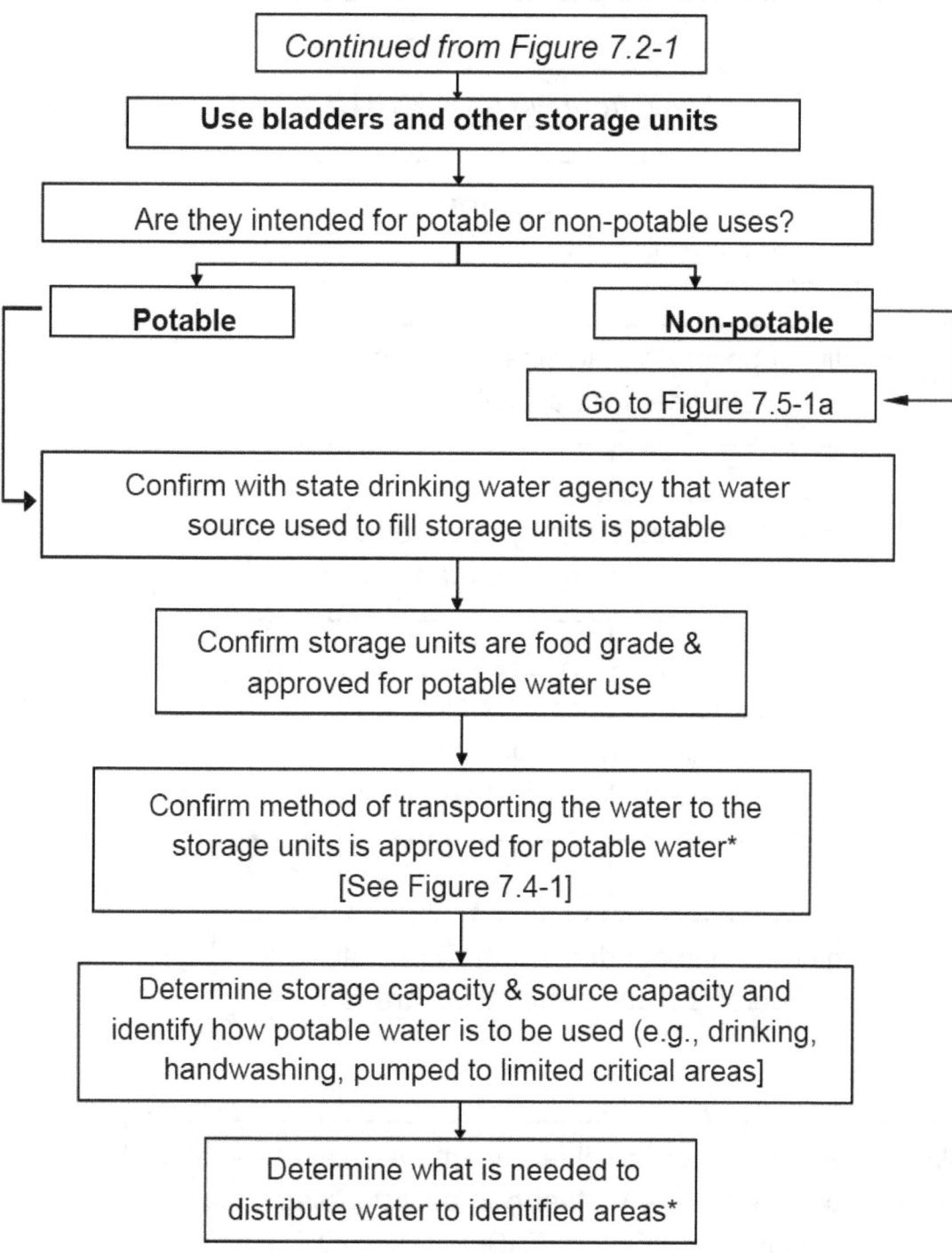

Continued from Figure 7.2-1

Use bladders and other storage units

Are they intended for potable or non-potable uses?

Potable

Non-potable

Go to Figure 7.5-1a

Confirm with state drinking water agency that water source used to fill storage units is potable

Confirm storage units are food grade & approved for potable water use

Confirm method of transporting the water to the storage units is approved for potable water*
[See Figure 7.4-1]

Determine storage capacity & source capacity and identify how potable water is to be used (e.g., drinking, handwashing, pumped to limited critical areas]

Determine what is needed to distribute water to identified areas*

*Do not use fire trucks for potable water pumping

Figure 7.5-1a

ALTERNATIVE WATER SUPPLIES - BLADDERS AND OTHER STORAGE UNITS FOR NON-POTABLE USES

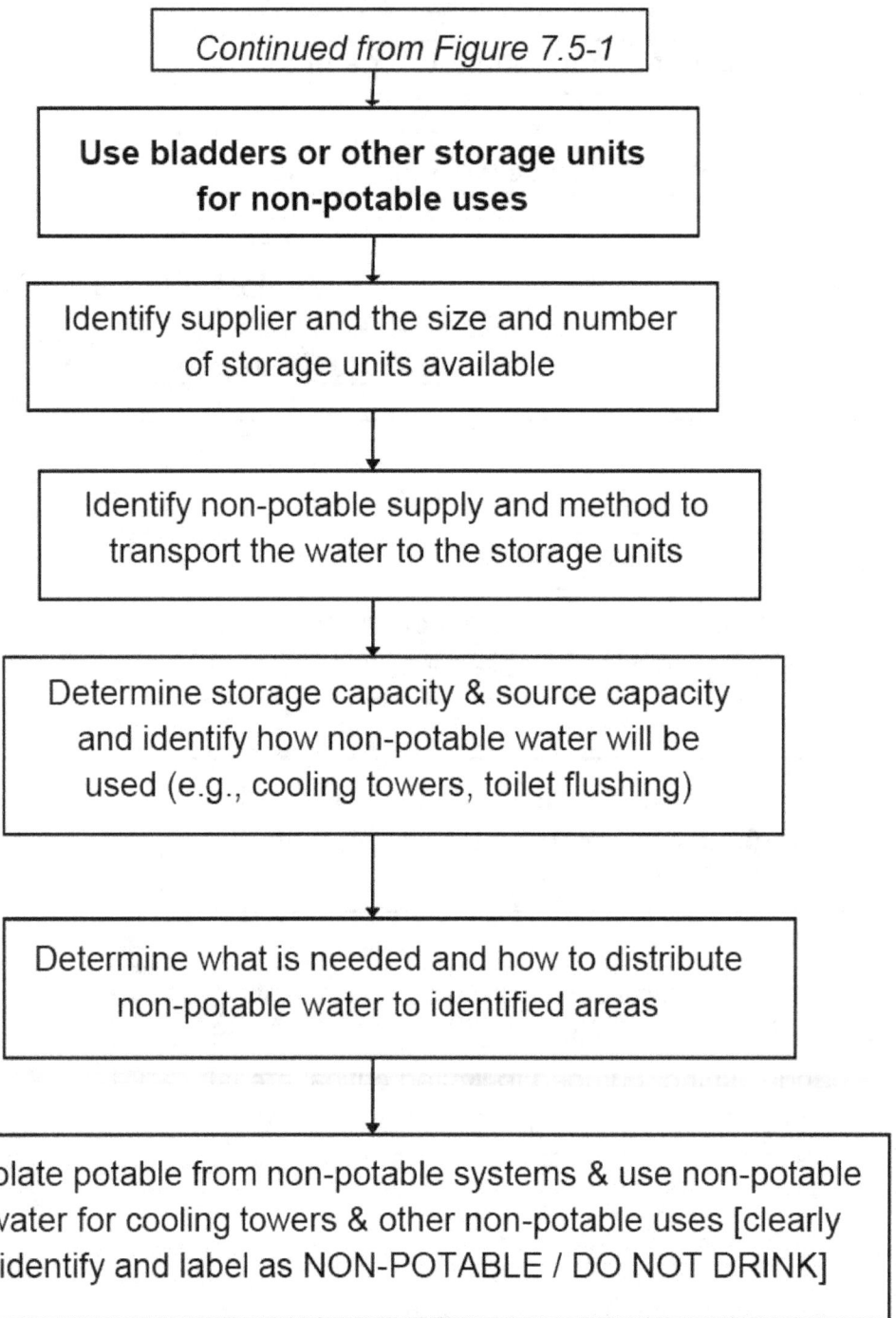

Figure 7.5-2. Pillow tanks

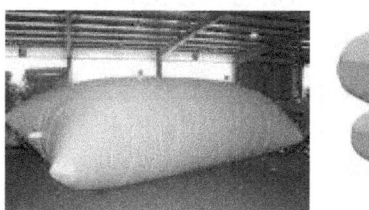 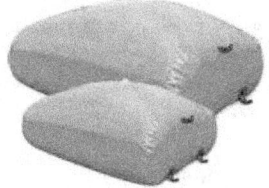

Figure 7.5-3. Bladder tanks

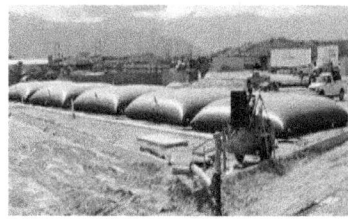 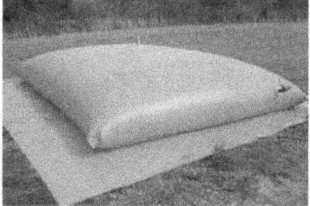

Figure 7.5-4. Onion water tank with removable cover

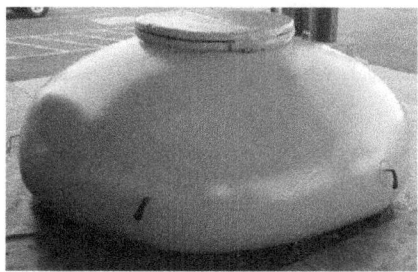

Figure 7.5-5. Pickup truck tank

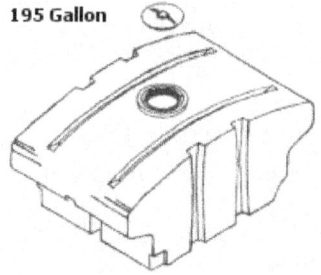

7.6. Water Storage Containers (55 Gallons and Smaller)

If emergency water storage is required on individual floors of a facility, smaller containers can be used. For planning purposes, consider the location and weight of the container when filled (Table 7.6-1). Depending on location and intended use, containers larger than 7 gallons may not be suitable because they would be too heavy for an individual to lift.

Table 7.6-1. Approximate Weight of Water-filled Containers

Container Size	Approximate Weight (in U.S. Pounds)
55 gallons	440 pounds
15 gallons	120 pounds
7 gallons	56 pounds
6 gallons	48 pounds
5 gallons	40 pounds
4 gallons	32 pounds
3 gallons	24 pounds
2 gallons	16 pounds
1 gallon	8 pounds

7.6.1. Storage Drums

If a large amount of water is needed on specific floors or sections, a 55-gallon food grade drum can be used (Figure 7.6-1). It should be placed out of the way and where the floor structure can support its weight when full (e.g., over 400 pounds).

A siphon or transfer pump can be used to dispense the water from the large container. Food-grade tubing should be used for siphoning.

For convenience and to minimize the risk of spilling water, a hand-operated transfer pump (Figure 7.6-2) can be used. Battery- and electric-operated pumps are available through retailers. A limitation is that batteries or electricity may not be available during or after a disaster.

7.6.2. Handled Jugs (3-5 Gallons) and Other Small Containers

Handled jugs come in 3-gallon (approx. 11.4 liters) and 5-gallon (approx. 18.9 liters) sizes (Figure 7.6-3). A hand-operated pump can be used to dispense water from such containers.

Bottles and containers made from hard clear or color tinted PETE plastic (i.e., recycling code 1) are preferred because the 1-gallon and 2.5-gallon milky white plastic jugs and containers made from soft HDPE plastic (i.e., recycling code 2) puncture easily or, if dropped, can open.

7.6.3. Treatment of Container-stored Water

Non-commercially-bottled stored water in filled containers should be treated with chlorine or other approved method in order to maintain a detectable free chlorine residual and prevent microbial growth during storage. When using non-commercially-bottled stored water during an emergency or other water interruption, the stored water should be tested at least daily to ensure an adequate chlorine residual is maintained. Information about preparing and storing a small emergency water supply can be found at: http://www.cdc.gov/healthywater/emergency/safe_water/personal.html .

7.6.4. Commercially Bottled Water

Commercially bottled water may provide the most convenient immediate source of potable water for use during an emergency. Several advantages of commercially bottled water include: a readily available source of contingency water during unforeseen emergencies, and an available higher level of water treatment (e.g., reverse osmosis, distillation) that may not be standard for tap water. However, a careful and knowledgable review of a commercial bottler's treatment methods is necessary to ensure adequate removal of pathogens and other contaminants of concern. A disadvantage of commercially bottled water is that it cannot be made available in quantities large enough to meet all hospital needs without becoming cost-prohibitive.

The CDC website has links to resources that instruct consumers on how to obtain further information about bottled water manufacturers' treatment methods. http://www.cdc.gov/healthywater/drinking/bottled/. The CDC also provides guidance for immunocompromised individuals in the form of a guide entitled: Cryptosporidiosis: A Guide to Commercially-Bottled Water and Other Beverages. http://www.cdc.gov/crypto/gen_info/bottled.html .

Facilities should make formal arrangements in advance with bottlers and bulk suppliers to ensure availability and delivery of a sufficient supply of bottled water during an emergency. Local suppliers may not be able to provide an adequate supply during a crisis.

See Section 7.7, Water Storage Location and Rotation, for information about storing bottled water.

Figure 7.6-1. 55-gallon Water Drum

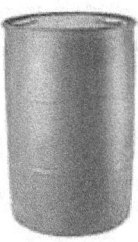

Figure 7.6-2. Hand Pump

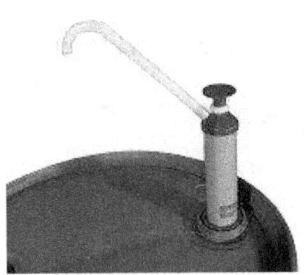

Figure 7.6-3. 3- and 5-gallon Containers

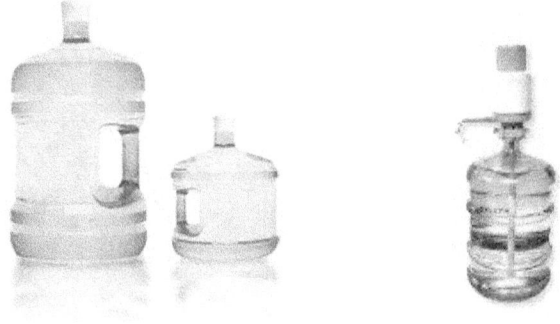

7.7. Water Storage Location and Rotation

All stored water should be kept in a cool dry place, out of direct sunlight, and, preferably, in a location not subject to freezing. Water containers should be stacked no higher than recommended by the manufacturer. If a large amount of water is stored, the structure of the floor must be sufficiently sound to support the weight of the water.

The American Red Cross and the Federal Emergency Management Agency recommend changing bottled water every 6 months. In the United States, commercially-bottled water manufacturers often mark a "sell by" date of 2 years after bottling. This "sell by" date serves as a stock-keeping number and for stock rotation purposes in supermarkets; it does not imply that the product is compromised or that water quality deteriorates after that date.

Health care facilities should ensure that the bottled water:

- is packaged in accordance with FDA processing and good manufacturing practices (21 CFR Part 129); http://www.accessdata.fda.gov/scripts/cdrh/cfdocs/cfcfr/CFRSearch.cfm?CFRPart=129 .
- meets FDA quality standard provisions as outlined in 21 CFR, Part 165; http://www.accessdata.fda.gov/scripts/cdrh/cfdocs/cfcfr/CFRSearch.cfm?CFRPart=165&showFR=1%20l
- meets standards for the removal of *Cryptosporidium* if used by immune compromised patients who are at risk for severe infection from this organism. More information is available in CDC's, *Guidelines for Preventing Opportunistic Infections Among Hematopoietic Stem Cell Transplant Recipients (2000)*; http://www.cdc.gov/mmwr/PDF/rr/rr4910.pdf
- has not been opened.

Tap water or water from other sources that is placed in containers and disinfected onsite (i.e. not commercially bottled) does not have an indefinite shelf life. Such water should be checked periodically for residual chlorine and retreated if necessary. See Section 7.6.3, Treatment of Container-stored Water, for additional information about non-commercially bottled water.

7.8. Portable Treatment Units

Water at facilities is used in both potable and non-potable applications. To keep the facility operational during an interruption of the public water supply, both needs have to be met in terms of quality and quantity. Many types of portable treatment technologies for meeting the water needs of facilities exist (See Section 7.10). However, the use of such technologies can be an expensive and complex process and generally is not recommended. If a portable treatment unit is used as an emergency water supply alternative, the monitoring requirements are typically complex and a certified treatment operator may be needed. Such a treatment unit should be pilot tested using the raw water source in order to assure operability and to provide hands-on operational experience for personnel who are expected to operate the equipment.

The choice of the type and size of treatment unit will depend on the available alternative water source and the intended use of the treated water. Figures 7.10-1 through 7.10-1d illustrate the steps to take when considering the use of portable treatment units. These efforts will require consultation with the state drinking water primacy agencies (http://www.epa.gov/safewater/dwinfo/index.html and http://www.asdwa.org/index.cfm?fuseaction=Page.viewPage&pageId=487).

7.8.1. Available Raw Water Sources

Raw water sources include surface water (e.g., rivers, lakes) and groundwater (e.g., wells). Surface water is more vulnerable to contamination both from point sources (e.g., sewage treatment plants, industrial plants, livestock facilities, landfills) and non point sources (e.g., septic systems, agriculture, construction, grazing, forestry, domestic and wildlife animals, recreational activities, careless household chemical management, lawn care, parking lot and other urban runoff).

During an emergency, it is not always possible to draw raw water from the pristine sources that supply the public water system and that have been thoroughly assessed under the Source Water Assessment and Protection Program. Source water might have to be drawn from streams, ponds, and shallow wells where water quality and susceptibility to contamination are unknown, but likely. Consultation with the state drinking water agency is critical to identify water quality parameters of concern in the source water to be used.

7.9. Contaminants: Biological and Chemical

Acute exposure to water contaminants is of primary concern during a reduction or complete loss of water pressure. Such fluctuations of pressure within a water distribution system can create a significant public health risks by causing:

- high intensity fluid shear with resultant resuspension of settled particles and/or biofilm detachment;
- intrusion of contaminated groundwater into pipes with cracks or leaky joints;
- entry of pathogens or other contaminants into the water distribution system because of improperly designed or maintained air relief valves or air chambers; and,
- chemical and/or biological contamination resulting from backsiphonage through unprotected faucets or failed/improperly maintained back-flow prevention devices.

To help detect potential chemical contamination, monitoring the water for any unusual tastes or odors should be instituted. A large intrusion of pathogens can cause the chlorine residual that normally is sustained in a drinking water distribution system to become insufficient to disinfect contaminated water, thus leading to potential adverse health effects.

In addition, heightened disease surveillance should be instituted to detect disease or illness that could be due to potential deterioration of the water quality.

7.10. Treatment Technologies

This section's listing of treatment technologies, their corresponding effectiveness for microbial contaminant removal or inactivation, and discussion of advantages and limitations is adapted from the National Environmental Service Center Tech Brief fact sheets series (National Environmental Service Center undated; http://www.nesc.wvu.edu/techbrief.cfm).

These treatment technologies are available as point-of-use (POU) systems for use at individual sinks or faucets, point-of-entry (POE) systems for use where water enters a building or structure, or as prepackaged treatment plants for large-scale water treatment of an entire health care facility complex.

The effectiveness of most filtration methods presented in Table 7.10-1 is impacted by the quality of the raw source water being treated. Typically, at a minimum, raw water is passed through cartridge filters before the more advanced reverse osmosis (RO) membrane treatment.

NSF/ANSI Drinking Water Treatment Unit (DWTU) Standards covering POU and POE technologies with respect to microbiological treatment include the following (http://www.nsf.org/business/drinking_water_treatment/standards.asp):

- **NSF/ANSI Standard 53**: Drinking Water Treatment Units - Health Effects
  Overview: Standard 53 addresses POU and POE systems designed to reduce specific health-related contaminants, such as *Cryptosporidium, Giardia*, lead, volatile organic chemicals (VOCs), MTBE (methyl tertiary-butyl ether), that may be present in public or private drinking water.
- **NSF/ANSI Standard 55:** Ultraviolet (UV) Microbiological Water Treatment Systems
  Overview: Standard 55 establishes requirements for POU and POE non-public water supply (non-PWS) UV systems and includes two optional classifications. Class A systems (40,000 μw-sec/cm^2) are designed to disinfect and/or remove microorganisms from contaminated water, including bacteria and viruses, to a safe level. Class B systems (16,000 μw-sec/cm^2) are designed for supplemental bactericidal treatment of public drinking water or other drinking water, which has been deemed acceptable by a local health agency.
- **NSF/ANSI Standard 58**: Reverse Osmosis (RO) Drinking Water Treatment Systems
  Overview: Standard 58 was developed for POU RO treatment systems. These systems typically consist of a prefilter, RO membrane, and post-filter. Standard 58 includes contaminant reduction claims commonly treated using RO, including fluoride, hexavalent and trivalent chromium, total dissolved solids, nitrates, etc. that may be present in public or private drinking water.
- **NSF/ANSI Standard 62**: Drinking Water Distillation Systems
  Overview: Standard 62 covers distillation systems designed to reduce specific contaminants, including total arsenic, chromium, mercury, nitrate/nitrite, and microorganisms from public and private water supplies.
- **NSF Protocol P231**: Microbiological Water Purifiers
  Overview: Protocol P231 addresses systems that use chemical, mechanical, and/or physical technologies to filter and treat waters of unknown microbiological quality, but that are presumed to be potable.

The state drinking water agency should be contacted to determine any certification requirements necessary to operate and use specific treatment devices.

To achieve a 3-log *Cryptosporidium* removal as recommended in CDC guidance, small-scale POU/POE treatment unit(s) using one or a combination of the filtration technologies should conform to specific package and labeling information (http://www.cdc.gov/parasites/crypto/gen_info/filters.html).

7.10.1. Disinfection

Boiling untreated water is not practical at the scale required to meet water needs for hospitals and outpatient facilities (e.g., ambulatory surgical-centers, dialysis centers, gastroenterology centers, urgent care centers). Complementary primary and secondary disinfection is recommended to enhance treatment reliability. Typically, microbial inactivation is improved in high-quality water (e.g., low turbidity, low organic matter). Elevated iron or manganese levels may require sequestration or physical removal for chlorine and ozone to work effectively. High organic matter and turbidity will impact the UV dose required for disinfection.

Table 7.10-1. Microbial Removal Achieved by Available Filtration Technologies

Unit technology	Limitations	Operator Skill Level Required	Raw Water Quality Range and Consideration	Removals: Log *Giardia* and Log Virus
Conventional Filtration (includes dual-stage and dissolved air flotation)	[Note A]	Advanced	Wide range of water quality. Dissolved air flotation is more applicable for removing particulate matter that doesn't readily settle: algae, high color, low turbidity—up to 30-50 nephelometric turbidity units (NTU) and low-density turbidity.	2-3 log *Giardia* and 1 log viruses
Direct Filtration (includes in-line)	[Note A]	Advanced	High quality. Suggested limits: average turbidity 10 NTU; maximum turbidity 20 NTU; 40 color units; algae on a case-by-case basis (National Research Council 1997)	0.5 log *Giardia* and 1-2 log viruses (1.5-2 log *Giardia* w/coagulation)
Slow Sand Filtration	[Note B]	Basic	Very high quality or pretreatment. Pretreatment required if raw water is high in turbidity, color, and/or algae.	4 log *Giardia* and 1-6 log viruses
Diatomaceous Earth Filtration	[Note C]	Intermediate	Very high quality or pretreatment. Pretreatment required if raw water is high in turbidity, color, and/or algae.	Very effective for *Giardia*; low bacteria and virus removal
Reverse Osmosis	[Notes D, E, F]	Advanced	Requires prefiltrations for surface water—may include removal of turbidity, iron, and/or manganese. Hardness and dissolved solids may also affect performance.	Very effective (cysts and viruses)
Nanofiltration	[Note E]	Intermediate	Very high quality of pretreatment. See reverse osmosis pretreatment.	Very effective (cysts and viruses)
Ultrafiltration	[Note G]	Basic	High quality or pretreatment	Very effective *Giardia*, >5-6 log
Microfiltration	[Note G]	Basic	High quality or pretreatment required.	Very effective *Giardia*, >5-6 log; partial removal viruses

(Continued)

Unit technology	Operator Skill Level Required	Limitations	Raw Water Quality Range and Consideration	Removals: Log *Giardia* and Log Virus
Bag Filtration	Basic	[Notes G, H, I]	Very high quality or pretreatment required because of low particulate loading capacity. Pretreatment if high turbidity or algae.	Variable *Giardia* removals and disinfection required for virus credit
Cartridge Filtration	Basic	[Notes G, H, I]	Very high quality or pretreatment required because of low particulate loading capacity. Pretreatment if high turbidity or algae.	Variable *Giardia* removals and disinfection required for virus credit
Backwashable Depth Filtration	Basic	[Notes G, H, I]	Very high quality or pretreatment required because of low particulate loading capacity. Pretreatment if high turbidity or algae.	Variable *Giardia* removals and disinfection required for virus credit

Notes on limitations of unit technology (Table 7.10-1):

A. Involves coagulation. Coagulation chemistry requires advanced operator skill and extensive monitoring. A system needs to have direct full-time access or full-time remote access to a skilled operator to use this technology properly.

B. Water service interruptions can occur during the periodic filter-to-waste cycle, which can last from 6 hours to 2 weeks.

C. Filter cake should be discarded if filtration is interrupted. For this reason, intermittent use is not practical. Recycling the filtered water can remove this potential problem.

D. Blending (combining treated water with untreated raw water) cannot be practiced at risk of increasing microbial concentration in finished water.

E. Post-disinfection recommended as a safety measure and for residual maintenance.

F. Post-treatment corrosion control will be needed before distribution.

G. Disinfection required for viral inactivation.

H. Site-specific pilot testing before installation likely to be needed to ensure adequate performance.

I. Technologies may be more applicable to system serving fewer than 3,300 people.

Figure 7.10-1

ALTERNATIVE WATER SUPPLIES - PORTABLE TREATMENT UNITS - *OVERVIEW*

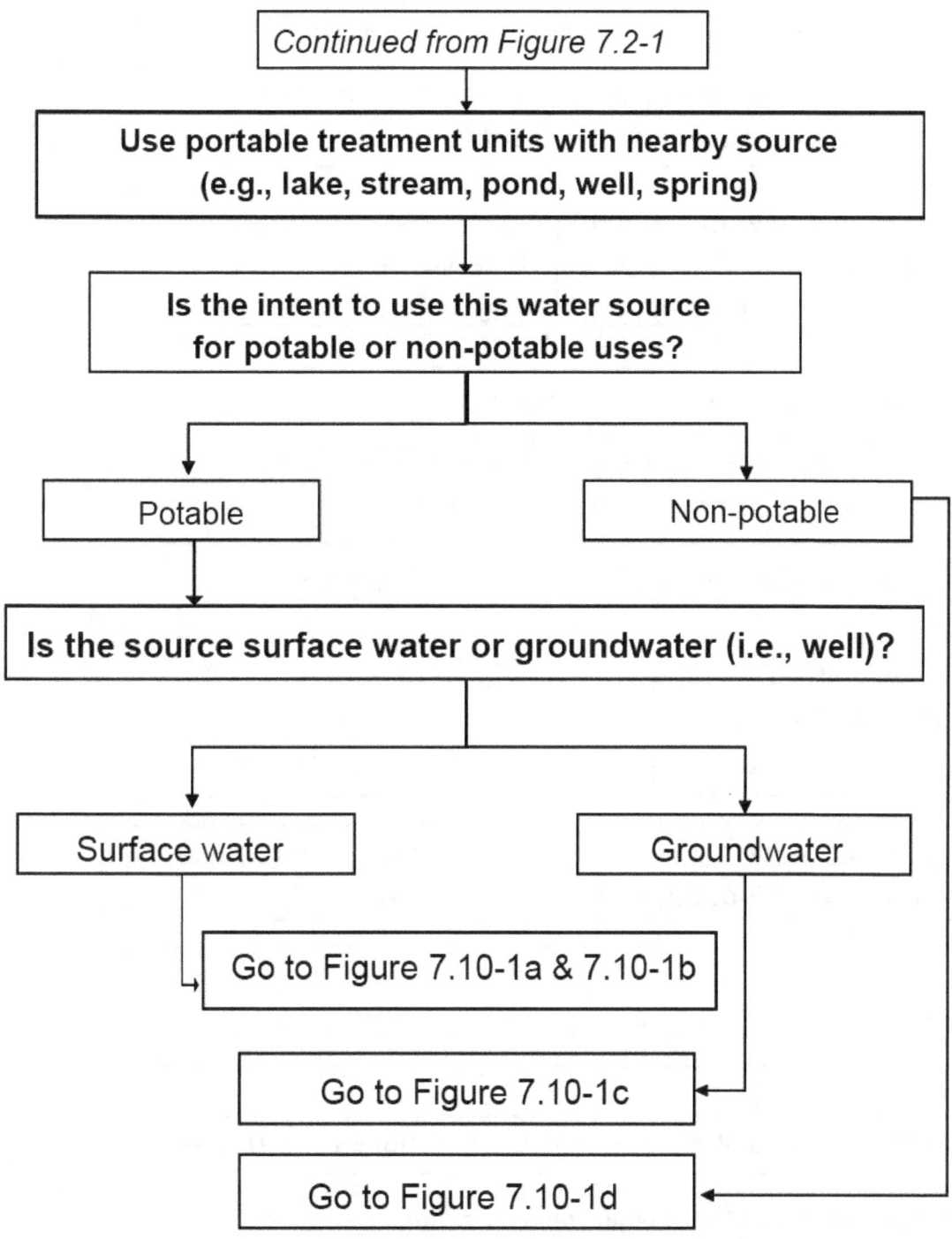

Figure 7.10-1a

ALTERNATIVE WATER SUPPLIES - PORTABLE TREATMENT UNITS FOR SURFACE WATER SOURCE

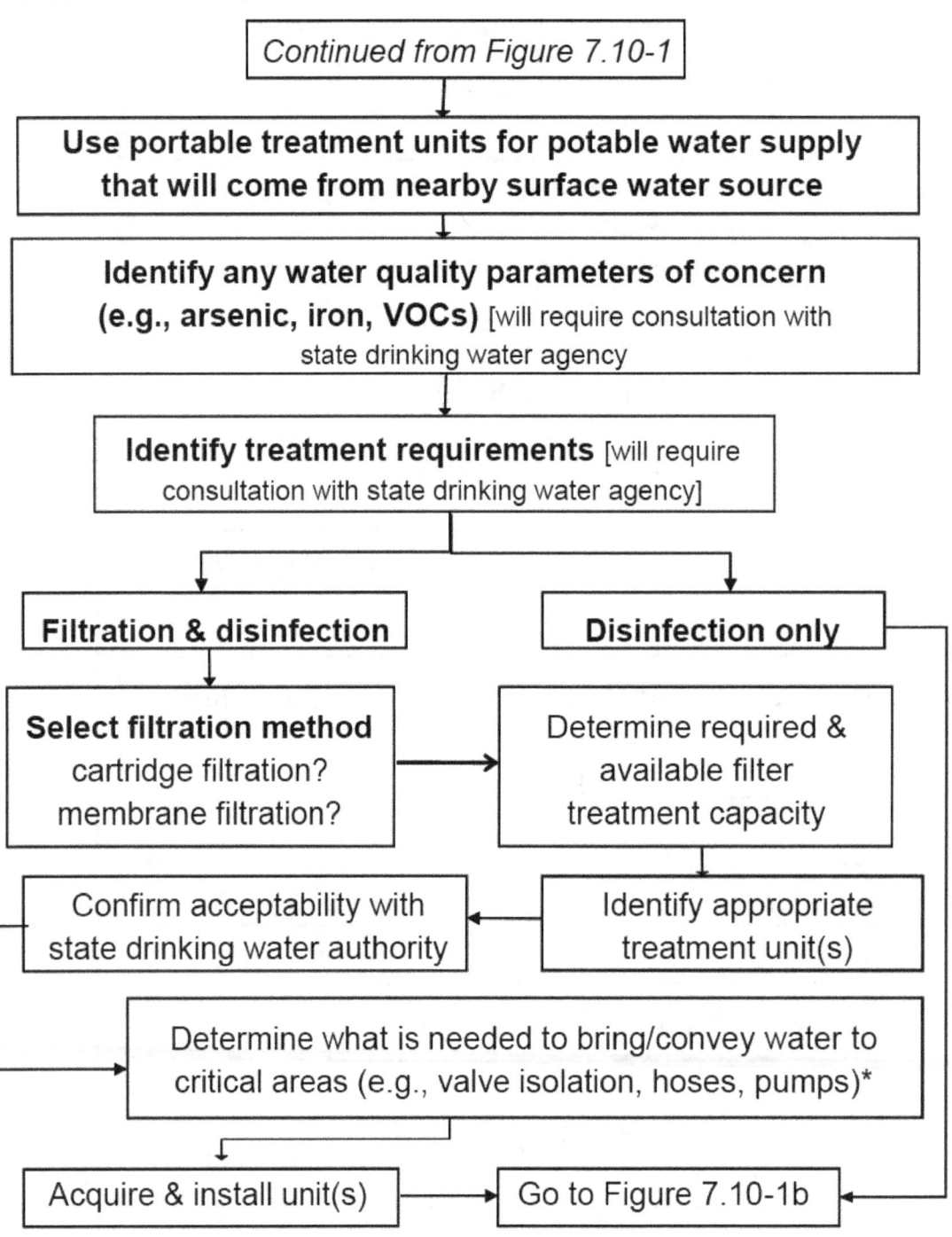

Do not use fire trucks for potable water pumping

Figure 7.10-1b
ALTERNATIVE WATER SUPPLIES - DISINFECTION OF SURFACE WATER

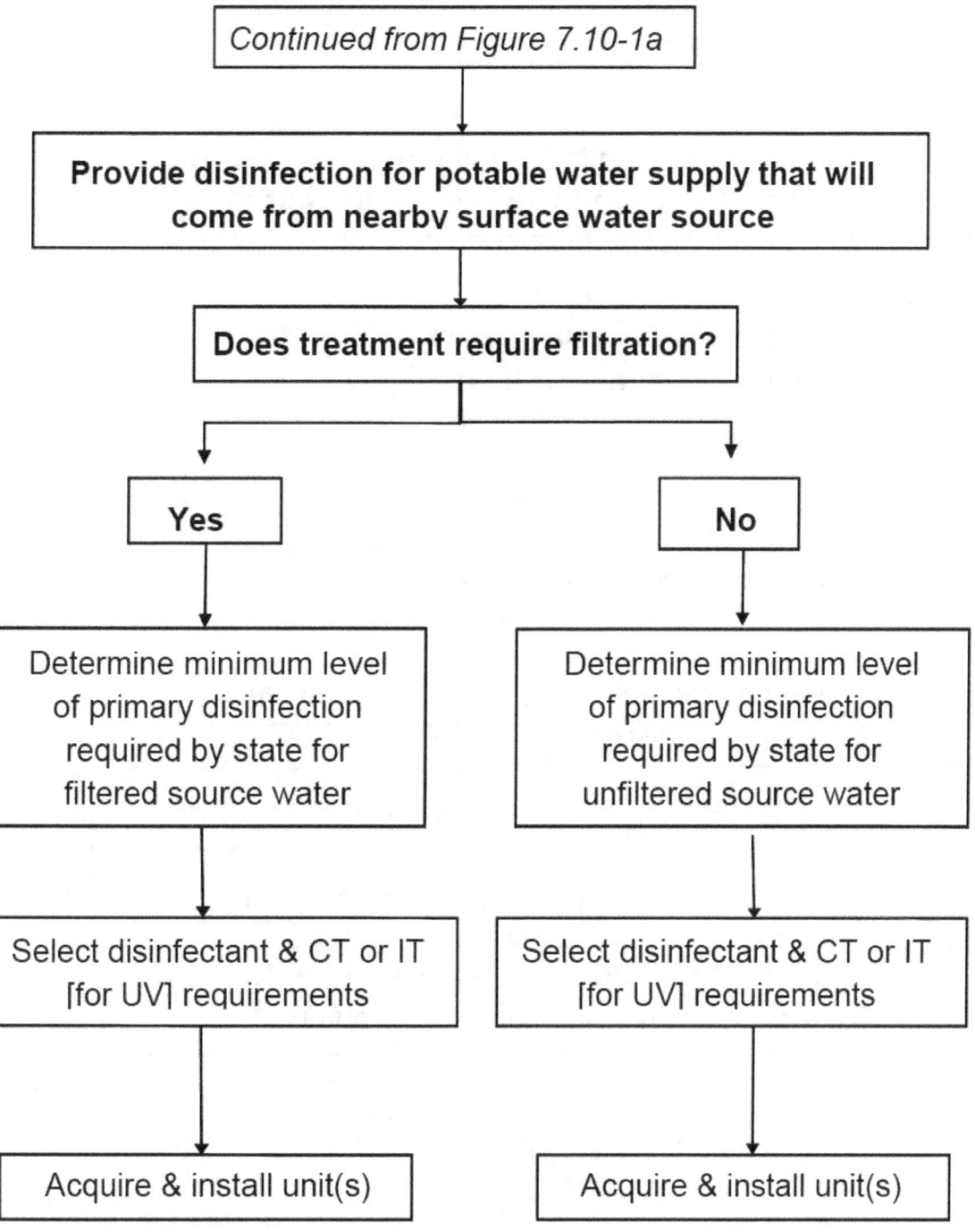

Continued from Figure 7.10-1a

Provide disinfection for potable water supply that will come from nearby surface water source

Does treatment require filtration?

Yes

No

Determine minimum level of primary disinfection required by state for filtered source water

Determine minimum level of primary disinfection required by state for unfiltered source water

Select disinfectant & CT or IT [for UV] requirements

Select disinfectant & CT or IT [for UV] requirements

Acquire & install unit(s)

Acquire & install unit(s)

Figure 7.10-1c

ALTERNATIVE WATER SUPPLIES - PORTABLE TREATMENT UNITS FOR GROUNDWATER SOURCE

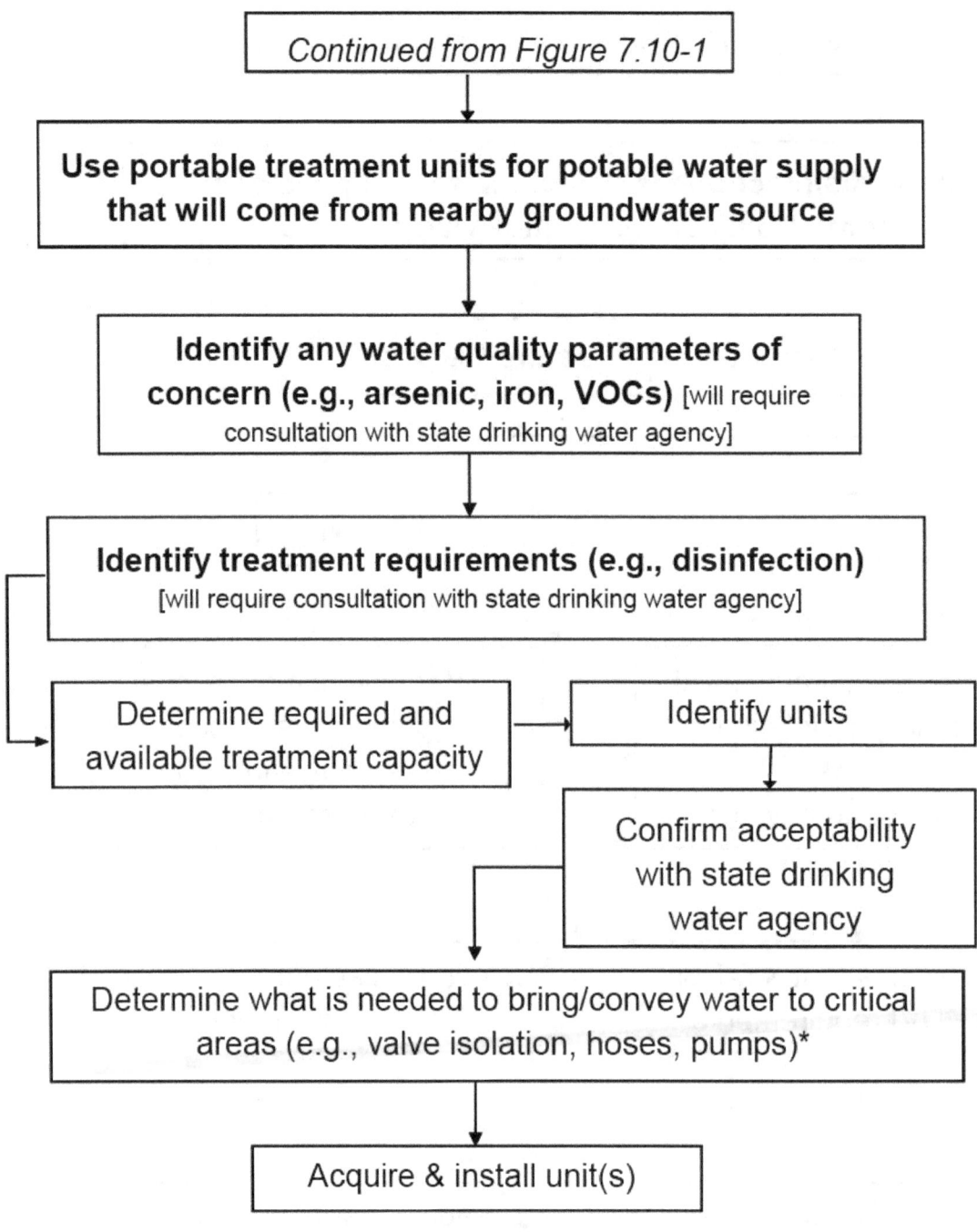

Continued from Figure 7.10-1

Use portable treatment units for potable water supply that will come from nearby groundwater source

Identify any water quality parameters of concern (e.g., arsenic, iron, VOCs) [will require consultation with state drinking water agency]

Identify treatment requirements (e.g., disinfection) [will require consultation with state drinking water agency]

Determine required and available treatment capacity

Identify units

Confirm acceptability with state drinking water agency

Determine what is needed to bring/convey water to critical areas (e.g., valve isolation, hoses, pumps)*

Acquire & install unit(s)

*Do not use fire trucks for potable water pumping

Figure 7.10-1d

ALTERNATIVE WATER SUPPLIES - PORTABLE TREATMENT UNITS FOR NON-POTABLE SUPPLY

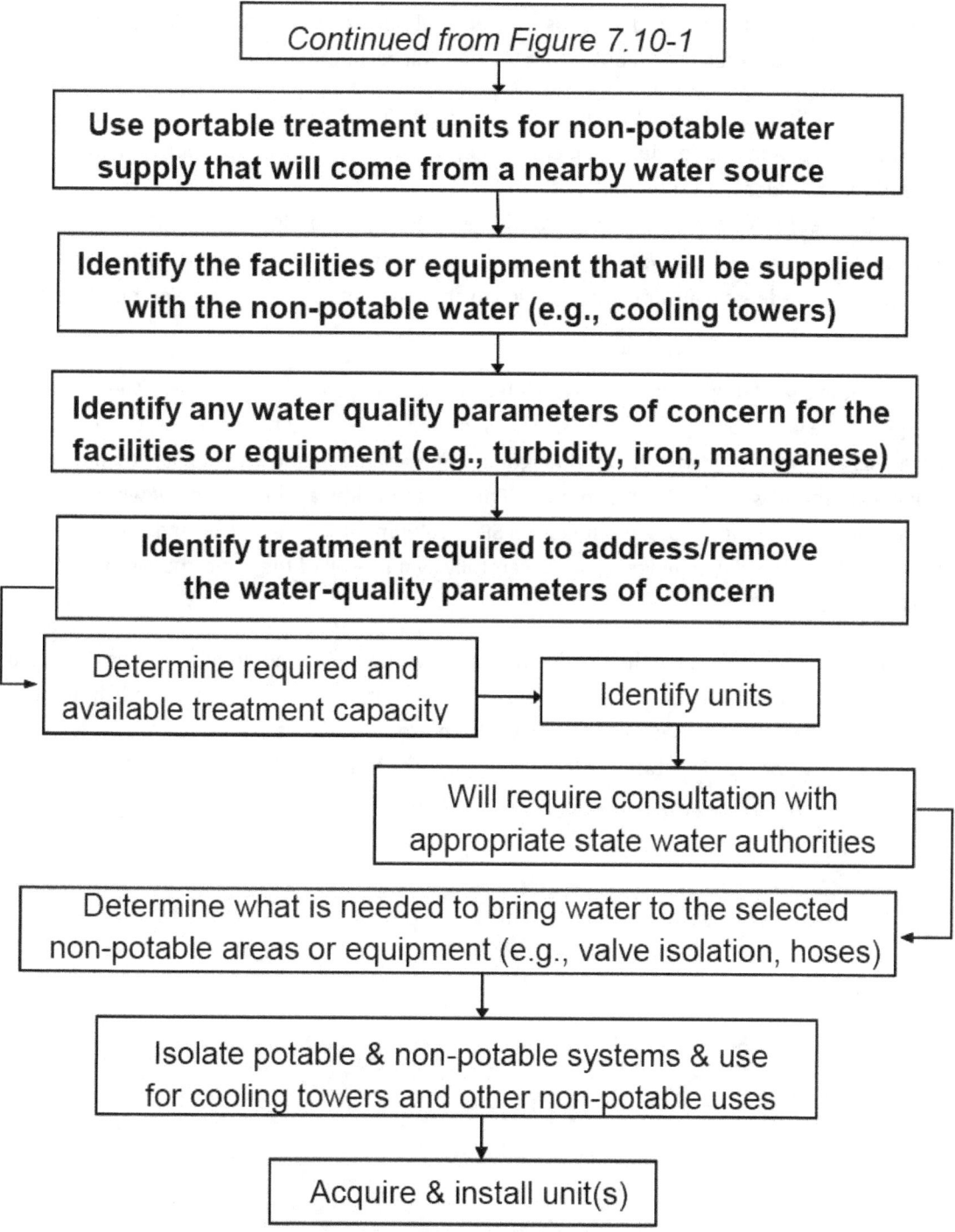

8. Conclusion

Health care facilities are a critical component to a community's recovery after a natural disaster, an accident, or an act of terrorism. The water supply for a facility could possibly be interrupted for any of these incidents. Health care facilities need to be prepared for a potential loss of their water supply in the same manner that that they are prepared for a loss of electrical power. It is not a question of whether the water supply will ever be interrupted, but rather when it will occur and for how long it will last.

The Joint Commission's Standard EM.02.02.09 (Joint Commission 2009) requires a critical access facility to address how it will manage utilities during an emergency as part of its EOP. As previously indicated, it is recommended that facilities not accredited by the Joint Commission also address emergency water supply planning. The Center for Medicare and Medicaid Services (CMS) Conditions for Participation/Conditions for Coverage (42 CFR 482.41) also requires that health care facilities make provisions in their preparedness plans for situations in which utility outages (e.g., gas, electric, water) may occur.

A key decision point in evaluating the incident and determining an appropriate response is the estimated length of the water outage. If the outage is estimated to last for 8 hours or less, the water supply alternatives are simpler. If the estimated length of the outage is unknown or longer than 8 hours, the water supply alternatives become more complex. For a large facility, a combination of water supply alternatives may be necessary for a longer outage. EWSP development is site-specific and should be based on local conditions. Facility managers should carefully evaluate all of these alternatives in finalizing their EWSPs.

Development of a written EWSP is only the starting point; the written plan should not be left sitting on a bookshelf. The EWSP should be a chapter in the overall facility emergency response plan and should be exercised on a regular basis and revised appropriately. These exercises can range from a relatively simple tabletop exercise with facility staff to a larger functional exercise involving appropriate outside agencies.

9. References

Agency for Healthcare Research and Quality. Hospital Evacuation Decision Guide. 2010 [cited December 20, 2010] Available from URL: http://www.ahrq.gov/prep/hospevacguide/.

Agency for Healthcare Research and Quality. Hospital Assessment and Recovery Guide. 2010 [cited December 20, 2010] Available from URL: http://www.ahrq.gov/prep/hosprecovery/

American Water Works Association. AWWA C652-02 standard for disinfection of water-storage facilities. Denver, CO: American National Standards Institute; 2002. [Cited 2010 Dec 2] Available from URL: http://www.techstreet.com/cgi-bin/detail?doc_no=AWWA|C652_02&product_id=961426

Beverages, 21 C.F.R. Sect. 165 (2009). [Cited 2010 Dec 1] Available from URL: http://www.accessdata.fda.gov/scripts/cdrh/cfdocs/cfcfr/CFRSearch.cfm?CFRPart=165&showFR=1%20l

CDC. Guidelines for preventing opportunistic infections among hematopoietic stem cell transplant recipients: recommendations of CDC, the Infectious Disease Society of America, and the American Society of Blood and Marrow Transplantation. MMWR 2000; 49:RR-10. [Cited 2010 Dec 2] Available from URL: http://www.cdc.gov/mmwr/preview/mmwrhtml/rr4910a1.htm.

Centers for Medicare and Medicaid Services. Emergency preparedness checklist. Survey and certification: emergency preparedness for every emergency. [Cited 2011 Jul 12] Available from URL: http://www.cms.gov/SurveyCertEmergPrep/downloads/S&C_EPChecklist_Provider.pdf

CDC. Commercially Bottled Water. [Cited 2010 Dec 2] Available from URL: http://www.cdc.gov/healthywater/drinking/bottled/.

CDC . Cryptosporidiosis: A Guide to Commercially-Bottled Water and Other Beverages. [Cited 2010 Dec 2] Available from URL: http://www.cdc.gov/crypto/gen_info/bottled.html.

Conditions of Participation for Hospitals, 42 C.F.R. Sect. 482.41– 482.42, 482.55. (2005). [Cited 2010 Dec 2] Available from URL: http://cfr.vlex.com/vid/482-condition-participation-physical-19811437.

Environmental Protection Agency. Guidance manual for compliance with the filtration and disinfection requirements for public water systems using surface water sources (570391001). Washington, DC: EPA; 1991. [Cited 2010 Dec 2] Available from URL: http://www.epa.gov/safewater/mdbp/guidsws.pdf.

Environmental Protection Agency. Source water assessment and protection program [online]. 2010. [cited 2010 Aug 17]. Available from URL: http://water.epa.gov/infrastructure/drinkingwater/sourcewater/protection/index.cfm .

Federal Emergency Management Agency. (2010). Water: how much water do I need? [online]. 2010. [Cited 2010 Aug 17]. Available from URL: http://www.fema.gov/plan/prepare/water.shtm.

Joint Commission. Approved: Revisions to emergency management standards for the critical access hospitals, hospitals, and long term care. Perspectives 2007;27(6):4,8. [Cited 2011 Jul 11]. Available from URL: http://www.naphs.org/documents/EmergencyMgtStandardsFinal.pdf.

Joint Commission. Emergency preparedness standards: utilities management (EM.02.02.09). Oakbrook Terrace, IL: Joint Commission; 2009.

National Environmental Service Center. Tech brief fact sheets [online]. 2010. [Cited 2010 Aug 17]. Available from URL: http://www.nesc.wvu.edu/techbrief.cfm.

NSF International. NSF protocol P231: microbiological water purifiers. Ann Arbor, MI: NSF International; 2003.[Cited 2010 Dec 2] Available from URL: http://www.techstreet.com/standards/NSF/P231_02_03?product_id=1082717.

NSF International. NSF/ANSI standard 53-2009e: drinking water treatment units - health effects overview. Ann Arbor, MI: NSF International; 2009. [Cited 2010 Dec 2] Available from URL: http://www.techstreet.com/cgi-bin/family?product_id=1650266.

NSF International. NSF/ANSI standard 55-2009: ultraviolet microbiological water treatment systems. Ann Arbor, MI: NSF International; 2009. [Cited 2010 Dec 2] Available from URL: http://www.techstreet.com/standards/NSF/55_2009?product_id=1648906.

NSF International. NSF/ANSI standard 58-2009: reverse osmosis drinking water treatment systems. Ann Arbor, MI: NSF International; 2009. [Cited 2010 Dec 2] Available from URL: http://www.techstreet.com/standards/NSF/58_2009?product_id=1648886.

NSF International. NSF/ANSI standard 60-2009: drinking water treatment chemicals. Ann Arbor, MI: NSF International; 2009. [Cited 2010 Dec 2] Available from URL: http://www.techstreet.com/standards/NSF/60_2009a?product_id=1701386.

NSF International. NSF/ANSI standard 61-2010a: drinking water system components. Ann Arbor, MI: NSF International; 2010. [Cited 2010 Dec 2] Available from URL: http://www.techstreet.com/standards/NSF/61_2010a?product_id=1752846.

NSF International. NSF/ANSI standard 62-2009: drinking water distillation systems. Ann Arbor, MI: NSF International; 2009. [Cited 2010 Dec 2] Available from URL: http://www.techstreet.com/standards/NSF/62_2009?product_id=1648866.

Processing and Bottling of Bottled Drinking Water, 21 C.F.R. Sect. 129 (2009). [Cited 2010 Dec 2] Available from URL: http://www.accessdata.fda.gov/scripts/cdrh/cfdocs/cfcfr/CFRSearch.cfm?CFRPart=129.

Well Construction and Pump Installation, Wisconsin Administrative Code NR 812.09(4)(a) (2002). [Cited 2010 Dec 2] Available from URL: http://dnr.wi.gov/org/water/dwg/forms/nr812.pdf.

Wisconsin Department of Commerce. Submittal information for review: health care facility water emergency supply. n.d. [cited 2010 Aug 17]. Available from URL: http://www.commerce. Available from URL: http://www.commerce.state.wi.us/sb/docs/SB-PlumbingHospitalWaterChecklist.pdf.

10. Bibliography

Adham SS, Jacangelo JG, Laine JM. Characteristics and costs of MF and UF plants. AWWA 1996;88:22–31. [Cited 2010 Dec 2]. Available from URL: http://www.awwa.org/publications/JournalCurrent.cfm.

American Nurses Association. Adapting standards of care under extreme conditions: guidance for professionals during disasters, pandemics, and other extreme emergencies [online]. 2008. [cited 2010 Aug 17]. Available from URL: http://nursingworld.org/MainMenuCategories/HealthcareandPolicyIssues/DPR/TheLawEthicsofDisasterResponse/AdaptingStandardsofCare.aspx.

American Water Works Association. Water chlorination and chloramination practices and principles. Manual of water supply practices M20. Denver, CO: AWWA; 2006. [Cited 2010 Dec 2] Available from URL: http://apps.awwa.org/EbusMain/Default.aspx?TabID=55&ProductId=6709.

American Water Works Association. Recommended practice for backflow prevention and cross-connection control. Manual of water supply practices M14. Denver, CO: AWWA; 2004 [Cited 2010 Dec 2] Available from URL: http://apps.awwa.org/EbusMain/Default.aspx?TabID=55&ProductId=6706.

California Association of Health Care Facilities. When disaster strikes [online]. n.d. [cited 2010 Mar 24]. Available from URL: http://www.cahf.org/DisasterPrep/PlanningGuidanceResources/DisasterPlanningforLTC/NursingHomeIncidentCommandSystemNHICS/tabid/351/Default.aspx.

California Emergency Medical Services Authority. Hospital incident command system (HICS) [online]. 2007. [cited 2010 Aug 17]. Available from URL: http://www.emsa.ca.gov/HICS.

Centers for Disease Control and Prevention. Disaster recovery information: Technical considerations when bringing hemodialysis facilities' water systems back on line after a disaster [online]. 2005. [cited 2010 March 24]. Available from URL: http://emergency.cdc.gov/disasters/watersystems.asp.

Centers for Disease Control and Prevention. Fact sheet: safe use of "tanker" water for dialysis [online]. 2005. [cited 2010 March 24]. Available from URL: http://emergency.cdc.gov/disasters/watertanker.asp.

Centers for Medicare and Medicaid Services. Emergency preparedness for dialysis facilities: a guide for chronic dialysis facilities [online]. 2005. [cited 2010 Mar 24]. Available from URL: http://www.cms.hhs.gov/esrdnetworkorganizations/downloads/emergencypreparednessforfacilities2.pdf.

Conditions for Coverage for End-Stage Renal Disease Facilities, 42 C.F.R. Sect. 405, 410, 413, 414, 488, and 494 2008. [Cited 2010 Dec 2] Available from URL: https://www.cms.gov/CFCsAndCoPs/13_ESRD.asp.

Environmental Protection Agency (US). EPA 816-F-06-027: Emergency disinfection of drinking water [online]. 2006. [cited 2010 Mar 24]. Available at http://www.epa.gov/safewater/faq/pdfs/fs_emergency-disinfection-drinkingwater-2006.pdf.

Environmental Protection Agency (US). EPA 816-F-09-004: National primary drinking water regulations [online]. 2009. [cited 2010 Mar 24]. Available from URL: http://www.epa.gov/ogwdw000/consumer/pdf/mcl.pdf.

Environmental Protection Agency (US). EPA 822-R-06-013: Drinking water standards and health advisories [online]. 2006. [cited 2010 Mar 24]. Available from URL: http://water.epa.gov/action/advisories/drinking/drinking_index.cfm.

Environmental Protection Agency. Guidance manual for compliance with the filtration and disinfection requirements for public water systems using surface water sources: EPA Number 570391001. Washington, DC: EPA; 1991. Available from URL: http://www.epa.gov/safewater/mdbp/guidsws.pdf.

Environmental Protection Agency (US). Guide standard and protocol for testing microbiological water purifiers. Washington, DC: U.S. Environmental Protection Agency; 1987. Available from URL: http://cfpub.epa.gov/ols/catalog/catalog_display.cfm?&FIELD1=SUBJECT&INPUT1=WATER%20PURIFICA TION%20EQUIPMENT%20%7BAND%7D%20SUPPLIES&TYPE1=EXACT&item_count=23.

Environmental Protection Agency (US). What are the health effects of contaminants in drinking water? [online]. 2004. [cited 2010 Mar 24]. Available from URL: http://permanent.access.gpo.gov/lps21800/www.epa.gov/safewater/dwh/health.html.

Federal Emergency Management Agency. Incident Command System (ICS) review material [online]. n.d. [cited 2010 March 24]. Available from URL: http://training.fema.gov/EMIWeb/IS/ICSResource/assets/reviewMaterials.pdf.

Federal Emergency Management Agency. IS 100.HC introduction to the incident command system for healthcare/hospitals [online]. 2007. [cited 2010 March 24]. Available from URL: http://training.fema.gov/EMIWeb/IS/is100HCb.asp.

Federal Emergency Management Agency. IS-200.a ICS for single resources and initial action incidents [online]. 2008. [cited 2010 March 24]. Available from URL: http://training.fema.gov/EMILMS/IS200a/index.htm.

Federal Emergency Management Agency. IS-700.a NIMS an introduction [online]. 2010. [cited 2010 March 24]. Available from URL: http://training.fema.gov/emiweb/is/is700a.asp.

Florida Health Care Association. Nursing home incident command system. n.d. [cited 2010 Mar 24]. Available from URL: http://www.fhca.org/emerprep/ics.php.

Food and Drug Administration. Reopening dialysis clinics after restoration of power and water. 2009. [cited 2010 Mar 24]. Available from URL: http://www.fda.gov/MedicalDevices/Safety/EmergencySituations/ucm055976.htm.

National Research Council Committee on Small Water Supply Systems. Safe water from every tap: improving water service to small communities. Washington, DC: National Academies Press; 1997. [Cited 2010 Dec 2] Available from URL: http://books.nap.edu/openbook.php?record_id=5291&page=1.

Navy Bureau of Medicine and Surgery. Water supply ashore: NAVMED P-5010-5. In: Manual of naval preventive medicine. Washington, DC: Bureau of Medicine and Surgery; 2008. Available from URL: http://www.med.navy.mil/directives/Pub/5010-5.pdf.

Sehulster LM, Chinn RYW, Arduino MJ, Carpenter J, Donlan R, Ashford D, et al. Guidelines for environmental infection control in health care facilities. Guidelines for environmental infection control in health-care facilities. Recommendations from CDC and the Healthcare Infection Control Practices Advisory Committee (HICPAC) [online]. 2003. [cited 2010 Mar 24]. Available from URL: http://www.cdc.gov/hicpac/pdf/guidelines/eic_in_HCF_03.pdf.

Water Research Foundation. Maintaining water quality in finished water storage facilities [online]. 1999. [cited 2010 Aug 17]. Available from URL: http://www.waterrf.org/Search/Detail.aspx?Type=2&PID=254&OID=90763.

Welter G, Bieber S, Bonnaffon H, DeGuida N, Socher M. Cross-sector emergency planning for water providers and healthcare facilities. Journal AWWA 2010;10(1):68-78. [Cited 2011 Jul 11]. Available from URL: http://www.obg.com/media/documents/2011/5/JAWWA_Paper_GregWelter.pdf.

Appendix A: Case Studies

Case Study No. 1: Large Academic Medical Facility

Located in the Southeastern United States, this 1.2-million-square-foot academic medical center has over 700 beds, 500 medical staff, 1,300 nurses, and 4,300 employees. In September 1999, Hurricane Floyd caused the worst flooding in the history of North Carolina. Electrical and water supplies were disrupted—the water supply for 4 days. Generators were used for most of the facility but the power was not sufficient for all air-conditioning needs. Only essential chillers were used and power was rotated. However, temperatures became uncomfortable in the hospital.

Because the fire suppression sprinkler system was down, there was a need to post fire watches throughout the complex. All elective surgeries were canceled; only emergency surgeries were carried out. Staff used dry hand washing and only sponge baths were available for patients. Food preparation was limited to simple items (e.g., sandwiches), and, because dishwashing was not available, disposable plates and utensils (e.g., paper, plastic) were used. Much of the material/supplies were bought from local establishments. There is no laundry service onsite and the contract laundry was able to maintain a limited supply of water. They maximized the use of packaged sterile supplies to minimize the use of sterilizers.

With respect to the water supply,

- "DO NOT DRINK" signs were posted in both English and Spanish.
- Bottled water was used for drinking and for limited food preparation. One-liter and 5-gallon bottles of water and ice were brought in as well. Local soft-drink distributors brought in much of the water. There was no shortage.
- At the time of the hurricane, the hospital had a 300-gallons-per-minute (gpm) water demand.
- There was an existing well that had previously been used for HVAC chillers, but it had not been used in a long time.
- The facility had previously provided an external hook-up for an emergency water supply.
- The fire department provided three 2,000-gallon dump pools. Well water was pumped into the dump pools and a fire truck was used to pump water into the hospital through the external hook-up.
- Initially adequate pressure in the acute care facility could not be attained because 700 flush valves were open. Staff had to manually close the flush valves to get pressure in the system.
- The three 2,000-gallon dump pools containing the well water supply could not keep up with the demand. The facility switched to an 80,000-gallon rehab pool near the external hook-up and pumped the well water into the this pool, from which it was then pumped via the fire truck into the hospital. Neighboring systems also provided water via three 1,000-2,000 gallon U.S. Forest Service tanker/pumper trucks that also dumped their water into the rehab pool.
- A gas tank was dropped off to feed pumpers but caught fire one evening in a building adjacent to the children's hospital. This fire was extinguished without incident.

With respect to human waste,

- Neither bucket dumping into toilets nor "red bagging" was practical. Disposal of urine from catheter patients' bags even became an issue.
- Fifty portable toilets were brought in for staff use.
- Because handling of patient wastes became problematic, the facility's regular toilets had to be brought back on line in a slow, careful, and controlled manner, one section at a time, to make sure valves held.

After Hurricane Floyd,

- The facility is now a 1.5-million-square-foot hospital complex.
- A new well was drilled with 700-gpm capacity to run all of the hospital complex.
- The new well is equipped with a sodium hypochlorite chlorination system and hydropneumatic tank; disinfectant is piped into the system using a spool piece that is removed when not in use (photos on next page).
- Additional power generator capacity has been installed to run all of the medical complex.
- New buildings now are designed with stand-alone power and with emergency water supply hook-ups.
- Previous water cooled systems (e.g. vacuum suction) were converted to air cooled where possible.
- In the event of another disruption, the medical facility
  - Should have sufficient water/power to meet demands;
  - Will still cease nonessential functions; and
  - Will close off nonessential areas for water, power, and fire (e.g., auditoriums, sparsely used wings)

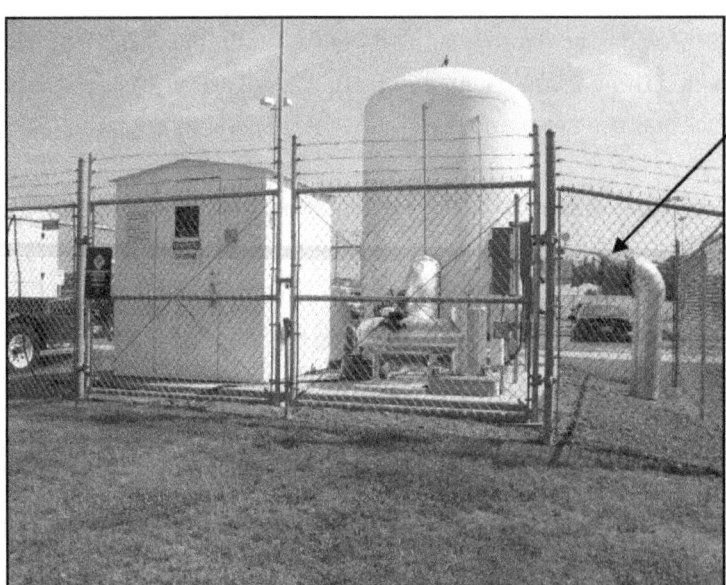

Spool piece to be removed when not in use

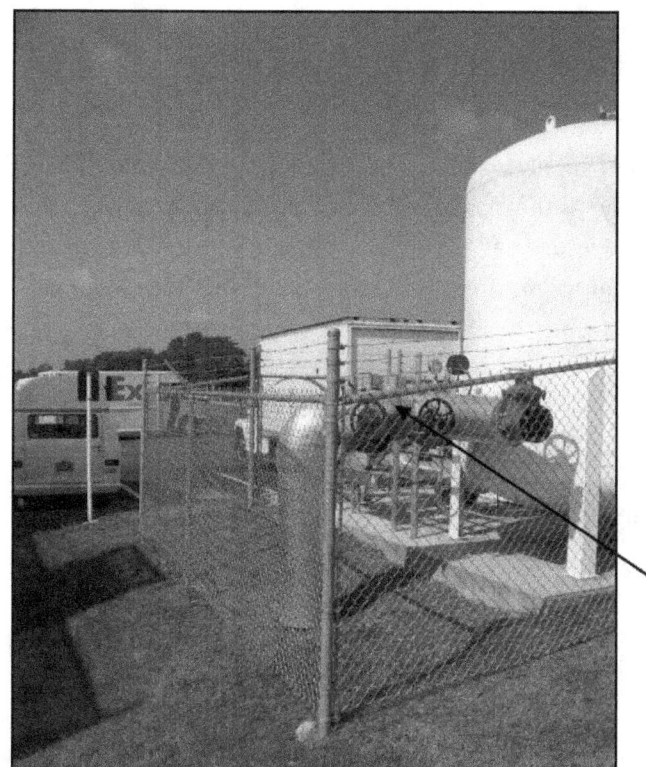

Spool piece

Case Study No. 2: Nursing Home

A 165-bed nursing home in Florida experienced a water supply interruption in 2004 because of Hurricane Ivan. As with most hurricanes, there were a few days to prepare before the hurricane made landfall. This facility stocked up on bottled water and other water containers and filled up every available container before landfall.

When the hurricane made landfall, the public water supply was interrupted because of a loss of power and the facility had to use the stocked water supply. As the loss of water service persisted through day one to day two, toilet flushing became a problem because each flush required a few gallons, rather than a few cups, of water, and the facility had shared bathrooms, thus preventing the option to wait longer between flushes.

As the loss of water service continued through day two to day three, facility staff went to the homes of staff who had swimming pools (which is relatively common in Florida) and filled up buckets and containers with pool water to bring back to the facility for toilet flushing. This effort was very labor-intensive (e.g. a gallon of water weighs more than 8 pounds) but it provided an adequate volume of water necessary for toilet flushing.

Appendix B: Example Plan

Introduction

The following is based on a project conducted at a 112-acre medical complex. This water use audit project was conceived after loss of the potable water supply following Hurricane Isabel in 2003. The storm surge and heavy rains caused flooding in the city, resulting in the loss of the potable water supply at the medical complex for about 4 days. Although the medical complex was able to secure a temporary water supply from an adjacent city via barges, it was recognized that this option might not be available during a future water supply interruption. Additionally, the staff noted that the existing emergency response plan for the medical complex lacked specific actions and water conservation strategies to implement during an emergency loss of the potable water supply.

Project Approach

This report addresses the following fundamental questions:

- In the event of a protracted and complete citywide water supply loss, what functions must remain in operation and what functions can be temporarily eliminated or substantially curtailed?
- How long can the critical functions in the acute-care facility (ACF) operate on the available stored water volume in the reservoir?
- What triggers the water conservation measures?

The ACF is the core-function facility at the medical complex. However, the staff identified specific support facilities as also critical to maintaining hospital functions in the ACF during a major emergency involving the loss of potable water supply. These facilities were included in the water use audit and are as follows:

- Medical support building: houses information technology functions, blood donation activity, refractive, and ambulatory surgery facilities
- Information technology buildings: houses information technology functions critical to patient care
- Central energy plant: includes large cooling towers that provide vital air chilling for the ACF

To address the above questions, the staff used the following approach:

- Supply only critical water use areas during a water supply outage
- Identify and estimate demands for the critical areas
- Determine actual water consumption for the entire medical complex, including annual averages and summer consumption (i.e. June, July, and August usage)
- Determine how long the medical complex can operate from the reservoir, without replenishment.

Water Use Audit Results

The project team performed staff interviews of each floor and department in the ACF to identify and estimate the critical area demands (i.e., the areas that should remain in service during a protracted water supply loss). Based on staff audits, departmental interviews, and the metering program, the following areas in the ACF were identified as critical:

- Sterilization
- Dining room
- Operating rooms
- Emergency room
- All laboratories
- Nephrology/dialysis
- Critical Care/Intensive Care Unit (ICU)
- Neonatal Intensive Care Unit (NICU)
- Gastroenterology clinic
- Post Anesthesia Care Unit (PACU)
- Compo B (complicated labor and delivery)
- Dental/oral maxifacial
- Critical Care Step Down Unit (SDU)
- Patient administrative computer services (PACS) computers.

Critical medical-related water demands include:

- Dialysis
- Sterilization and equipment washing
- Diagnostic equipment (e.g., MRI cooling water)
- Water seal for medical gas pumping (air, oxygen, nitrous oxide, vacuum)

Medical Complex Consumption

Knowing the average daily water consumption of the entire medical complex was necessary to estimate the length of time the facility could operate on its existing 2-million-gallon (MG) reservoir without water conservation restrictions. The annual average consumption and summer consumption in millions of gallons per day (MGD) for the entire complex are

- Annual average (2003-2008): 0.353 MGD
- Annual average (FY 2007): 0.366 MGD
- Summer average (June, July, August/ 2003-2008): 0.433 MGD.

Most of the complex's water demands are from the ACF and the central energy plant. Consequently, each of these buildings has a water meter on the cold water supply line entering the building. Based on meter readings, the average daily consumption of these facilities is

- ACF: 0.212 MGD (flow measured during study)

- Central energy plant (September 2006--December 2007): 0.157 MGD
- Central energy plant (July–August 2007): 0.212 MGD

Operating Duration of Reservoir During Water Outage

The existing 2-MG reservoir is typically kept at 84% full, or 1.68 MG. Table B-1 presents the time the medical complex can operate on the reservoir alone under different scenarios. As indicated in Table B-1, depending on the amount of water in the tank at the time of the interruption, for unrestricted water use, it can be estimated that the onsite storage tank can provide water for up to 4.6 days. Because the ACF and the central energy plant account for most of the water usage at this medical complex, limiting water use to these two buildings but not restricting water use within the ACF provides little increase in the amount of time that this medical complex could remain in operation. However, limiting water use to these two buildings and only to critical functions can result in water being available for up to 7.2 days depending on the water level in the tank.

Table B-1. Estimated Reservoir Operational Duration

Area Supplied With Water	Average Summer Consumption	Supply (Reservoir at 2 MG)	Supply (Reservoir at 1.68 MG)	Supply (Reservoir at 1 MG)	Supply (Reservoir at 0.5 MG)
Medical complex	0.433 MGD	4.6 days	3.9 days	2.3 days	1.2 days
ACF	0.210 MGD	9.5 days	8.0 days	4.8 days	2.4 days
Central energy plant	0.212 MGD	9.4 days	7.9 days	4.7 days	2.4 days
ACF & central energy plant	0.422 MGD	4.7 days	4.0 days	2.4 days	1.2 days
ACF critical areas & central energy plant	0.278 MGD	7.2 days	6.0 days	3.6 days	1.8 days

Recommended Response Plan for Water Outage

For this facility, temporary water conservation measures should be implemented if the water supply loss will likely last more than 24 hours, such as contamination from a natural disaster or a major water main break. These measures should include the following:

- Make advanced emergency preparations (if possible),
- Suspend nonessential services,
- Implement other water conservation measures,
- Isolate the water supply, and
- Activate Emergency Support Services.

Advanced Emergency Preparations

Maintain current reservoir operational practices, keeping the reservoir at 18.5 of 22 feet or higher whenever possible. In the event that a potential water emergency is identified (e.g., hurricanes being forecasted), the reservoir could be filled to 100% of storage capacity. Ensure water supply practices are in compliance with U.S. Environmental Protection Agency regulations and American Water Works Association (AWWA) standards.

If a storm event is anticipated, the medical complex should stock up on several essential items including:

- Fuel oil for power generation,
- Small backup generators (to provide redundancy) to operate pumps and other equipment,
- One reverse osmosis or nanofiltration skid that can provide one-half MGD of treated water,
- Emergency water disinfectant chemicals (e.g., bleach),
- Waterless hand sanitizer,
- Disposable sheets and pillow cases and covers because normal laundry service may not be available,
- Disposable sterile items such as catheters (i.e., to limit sterilization use),
- Water tanks on skids for water storage.

Nonessential Services

The following nonessential services can be suspended until normal water supply service is returned:

- Psychiatric services for patients needing limited care,
- All clinic services except nephrology, gastroenterology, pulmonary, internal medicine and infectious disease,
- Elective and non life-threatening surgeries,
- Physical therapy.

Other Water Conservation Measures

When possible, other water conservation measures should include use of waterless hand hygiene products (substitution should only be made when appropriate and in accordance with current infection control recommendations); sponge bathing patients; limiting food preparation to sandwiches or meals ready-to-eat (MREs); reducing dishwashing by using disposable plates, bowls, cups, and other eating utensils; restricting heating and cooling to essential buildings and to the essential areas within these buildings; closing nonessential areas (e.g., auditoriums) within essential buildings; and consolidating wings with a low patient population.

Isolation of Water Supply

An isolation plan was developed to provide water from the reservoir to the ACF and the central energy plant by using the shortest route and largest pipes possible to minimize flow restrictions. The isolation plan is summarized as follows:

1. Disconnect the medical complex from the city water supply,
2. Redirect flow to supply the ACF and the central energy plant first,
3. Isolate the remainder of the medical complex from the water supply system,

4. Further isolate noncritical areas within the ACF, if possible,

Specifically, the steps for isolating the medical complex's water supply are:

- Medical complex disconnection. To disconnect the medical complex from the city water supply in order to reduce the potential for contamination with city water: make sure that all valves at three locations of city water meters—downstream of the meter—are closed:
  - A1 (6 inch near reservoir)
  - D26 (6 inch main gate)
  - D21 (6 inch but may be a valve on 12-inch connection)
- Reservoir. To initiate water flow from the reservoir to the ACF and central energy plant, close the following valves:
  - A2: downstream of meter
  - A6 & A-8: isolates most of the complex
- Nonessential facilities. To isolate the rest of the medical complex from the central energy plant, close the following valves:
  - B6: Northwest feed to/from the central energy plant
  - A44: near the public works building—isolates the rest of the complex

5. Isolate the rest of the complex from the ACF by closing the following valves:
   - A22: isolates internal administration and School of Health Sciences
   - A23: isolates playing field, helipad, and gym
   - A24: isolates gym
   - A25: isolates temporary housing area no. 1
   - A51: isolates temporary housing area no. 2, convenience store, and swimming pool
   - A54: isolates convenience store
   - B3: isolates all buildings southwest of the ACF
   - B13: isolates executive administration building
   - B16: serves as backup to B13
   - D1: isolates all buildings south of ACF

The above valves should be positively located and confirmed to be in proper working order as part of a routine annual maintenance program. Closing valves A23, A24, A25, A51, and A54 is required to isolate the northern section of the complex. These steps could be eliminated and the water supply emergency response time could be greatly reduced by installing a single 8-inch valve in the existing pipe line along the main road north from the reservoir. Exercising (i.e. testing the operation of) these valves and testing this isolation plan before an emergency is highly recommended.

Restoring the medical complex to normal service after a water supply emergency would occur in the reverse sequence after the water distribution mains are disinfected in accordance with state and AWWA standards.

Emergency Support Services

Activate the standing contracts to provide the following emergency support services:

- Portable toilets,
- Instrument sterilization,
- Medical supplies,
- Meal preparation, and
- Potable water via truck or barge from the adjacent city.

Appendix C: Loss-of-Water-Scenario

The following scenario is a resource from the Hospital Incident Command System (HICS) website http://www.hicscenter.org/cods/215.swfv.

Health care facility staff who are involved, or may become involved, with emergency planning, response, and/or recovery efforts are encouraged to become familiar with HICS, the Incident Command System (ICS), and the National Incident Management System (NIMS). The Federal Emergency Management Agency (FEMA) recommends a series of online training courses by which health care facility staff can learn the basic concepts of the ICS, NIMS, and National Response Framework (e.g. IS-100, IS-200, IS-700, IS-800). Information about ICS, NIMS and HICS can be found at: http://www.fema.gov/emergency/nims/NIMSTrainingCourses.shtm and http://www.hicscenter.org/index.php .

Scenario

Without warning, the main water supply line to the hospital breaks, disrupting water service to the entire facility. The hospital's water systems, including potable water supply are nonfunctional. Local water sources and vendors are not impacted. Services, including food and radiology, are disrupted. Toilets and hand washing areas are not functioning and alternate methods must be provided

Utility workers expect to repair the damage and restore water service to the hospital within 10-12 hours.

Does Your Emergency Management Plan Address the Following Issues?

Mitigation & Preparedness

1. Does your hospital Emergency Management Plan include triggers or criteria for activation of the Emergency Operations plan and the Hospital Command Center?
2. Does your hospital have a plan for loss of water to the facility and sustaining operations?
3. Does your hospital have MOUs and/or contracts for provision of potable water?
4. Does your hospital have a process for determining the impacts of the loss of water on clinical operations (e.g., surgery schedule, outpatient services) and infrastructure systems?
5. Does your hospital have a plan and systems to connect to alternate water sources to support sprinkler system, waste water, and cooling systems?
6. Does your hospital have procedures to communicate situation and safety information to staff, patients, and families?
7. Does your hospital have procedures to evaluate the need for and to obtain additional staff?
8. Does your hospital have procedures to establish portable toilets and hand washing stations throughout the facility?
9. Does your hospital have a process to determine the need for partial or complete evacuation of the facility?
10. Does your hospital have a procedure for rationing potable water, if necessary?

11. Does your hospital have a plan for communicating water conservation measures to employees and patients?
12. Does your hospital have a plan to provide regular media briefings and updates?
13. Does your hospital have a plan to communicate with local emergency management and the water company about the situation and to request assistance?

Response and Recovery

1. Does your hospital have procedures for providing regular situation status updates to the local emergency management agency and water company?
2. Does your hospital have a process to evaluate the short and long-term impact of the loss of water on the patients, staff, and facility?
3. Does your hospital have a process to determine the need for canceling elective procedures and surgeries and other nonessential hospital services (e.g., gift shop) and activities (e.g., conferences, meetings)?
4. Does your hospital have criteria and a process to determine the need for complete or partial evacuation of the facility?
5. Does your hospital have a process to assess patients for early discharge to decrease patient census?
6. Does your hospital have a plan to provide staff with information on the situation and emergency and water conservation measures to implement?
7. Does your hospital have procedures to notify patients' family members of the situation?
8. Does your hospital have a process to cancel nonessential functions (e.g., meetings, conferences, gift shop)?
9. Does your hospital have a process to determine the need to limit patient visitation?
10. Does your hospital have a plan to document actions, decisions, and activities and to track response expenses and lost revenues?
11. Does your hospital have procedures to provide accurate and timely briefings to staff, patients, families, and area hospitals during extended operations?
12. Does your hospital plan for demobilization and system recovery during response?
13. Does your hospital have facility and departmental business continuity plans? Do these plans address the need for alternate service providers for critical hospital functions (e.g., radiology, laboratory)?
14. Does your hospital have a plan to conduct regular media briefings in collaboration with the local emergency management agency?
15. Does your hospital have procedures for restoring normal facility visitation and nonessential service operations (e.g., gift shop, conferences)?
16. Does your hospital have procedures for repatriation of patients who were transferred or evacuated?
17. Does your hospital have procedures for after-action reporting and development of an improvement plan?

Incident Response Guide

Mission: To effectively and efficiently manage the effects of a loss of water in the facility.

Directions

- ❑ Read this entire response guide and review the Incident Management Team Chart (Figure C.1). (Remember that the number of activated positions will increase as the response progresses.)
- ❑ Use this response guide as a checklist to ensure all tasks are addressed and completed.

Objectives

- ❑ Conserve water and restore water supply
- ❑ Identify and obtain alternate sources of potable water
- ❑ Maintain patient care management
- ❑ Monitor heating and cooling systems

IMMEDIATE (OPERATIONAL PERIOD 0-2 HOURS)

COMMAND STAFF

(Incident Commander):

- ❑ Activate the facility Emergency Operations Plan
- ❑ Activate Command Staff and Section Chiefs, as appropriate
- ❑ Establish incident objectives and operational period

(Liaison Officer):

- ❑ Notify local emergency management of hospital's situation status, critical issues, and timeline for water service repairs and restoration
- ❑ Notify the water utility and outside agencies of water loss and estimated time for water main repair and restoration of service
- ❑ Notify local EMS and ambulance providers about the situation and possible need to evacuate
- ❑ Communicate with other health care facilities to determine
    - ❑ Situation status
    - ❑ Surge capacity
    - ❑ Patient transfer/bed availability
    - ❑ Ability to loan needed equipment, supplies, medications, personnel, and other resources
- ❑ Contact the Regional Hospital Coordination Center, if one exists, to notify about the situation and request assistance with patient evacuation destinations

(Public Information Officer):

❏ Inform staff, patients, and families of situation and measures to conserve water and protect life

❏ Prepare media staging area

❏ Conduct regular media briefings in collaboration with local emergency management, as appropriate

(Safety Officer):

❏ Evaluate safety of patients, family, staff, and facility and recommend protective and corrective actions to recognize and minimize hazards and risks

OPERATIONS SECTION

❏ Determine impact of water loss on systems and patients

❏ Estimate potable and non-potable water usage and needs and collaborate with Logistics Section and Liaison Officer to obtain backup water supplies

❏ Access alternate sources of water to provide for fire suppression, HVAC system, and other critical systems, as able

❏ Institute rationing of water, as appropriate

❏ Initiate water conservation measures

❏ Assess patients for risk and prioritize care and resources, as appropriate

❏ Monitor infection control practices

❏ Provide alternate toilet and hand washing facilities

❏ Secure the facility and implement limited visitation policy

❏ Ensure continuation of patient care and essential services

❏ Consider partial or complete evacuation of the facility, or relocation of patients and services within the facility

❏ Activate the business continuity plans for the facility and impacted departments

PLANNING SECTION

❏ Establish operational periods and incident objectives, and develop the Incident Action Plan, in collaboration with the Incident Commander

❏ Prepare for patient and personnel tracking in the event of evacuations

LOGISTICS SECTION

❏ Maintain other utilities and activate alternate systems as needed

❏ Investigate and provide recommendations for alternate water supplies, including potable water

❏ Assist with rationing water, as appropriate

❏ Obtain supplemental staffing, as needed

❏ Prepare for transportation of patients, if evacuation plan is activated

❏ Oversee and conduct water main repairs and restoration of services

INTERMEDIATE AND EXTENDED (OPERATIONAL PERIOD 2 HOURS TO GREATER THAN 12 HOURS)

COMMAND STAFF

(Incident Commander):

- ❑ Update and revise the Incident Action Plan and prepare for demobilization
- ❑ Continue to update internal officials on the situation status
- ❑ Monitor evacuation

(PIO):

- ❑ Continue briefings and situation updates with staff, patients, and families
- ❑ Continue patient information center operations, in collaboration with Liaison Officer
- ❑ Assist with notification of patients' families about situation and transfer/evacuation, if activated

(Liaison Officer):

- ❑ Continue to notify local EOC of situation status and critical issues, and request assistance, as needed
- ❑ Continue to communicate with local utilities about incident details and estimated duration
- ❑ Continue patient information center operations, in collaboration with PIO
- ❑ Continue communications with area hospitals and facilitate patient transfers

(Safety Officer):

- ❑ Continue to evaluate facility operations for safety and hazards and take immediate corrective actions

OPERATIONS SECTION

- ❑ Continue evaluation of patients and patient care
- ❑ Cancel elective surgeries and procedures
- ❑ Prepare the staging area for patient transfer/evacuation
- ❑ Initiate ambulance diversion procedures
- ❑ Continue or implement patient evacuation
- ❑ Ensure the transfer of patients' belongings, medications, and records upon evacuation
- ❑ Continue to ration water, especially potable water, as appropriate
- ❑ Maintain facility security and restricted visitation
- ❑ Continue to maintain other utilities
- ❑ Monitor patients for adverse health effects and psychological stress
- ❑ Prepare demobilization and system recovery plan

PLANNING SECTION

- ❑ Continue patient, bed, and personnel tracking
- ❑ Update and revise the Incident Action Plan
- ❑ Prepare the demobilization and system recovery plans
- ❑ Plan for repatriation of patients
- ❑ Ensure documentation of actions, decisions, and activities

LOGISTICS SECTION

- ❑ Continue with nutritional, sanitation, and HVAC support and operations
- ❑ Contact vendors to provide emergency potable and non-potable water supplies and portable toilets
- ❑ Monitor the impact of the loss of water on critical areas
- ❑ Continue to provide staff for patient care and evacuation
- ❑ Monitor staff for adverse affects of heath and psychological stress
- ❑ Monitor, report, follow up on, and document staff or patient injuries
- ❑ Continue to provide transportation services for internal operations and patient evacuation

FINANCE/ADMINISTRATION SECTION

- ❑ Continue to track costs, expenditures, and lost revenue
- ❑ Continue to facilitate contracting for emergency repairs and other services

DEMOBILIZATION/SYSTEM RECOVERY

COMMAND STAFF

(Incident Commander):

- ❑ Determine hospital status and declare restoration of normal water services and termination of the incident
- ❑ Notify state licensing, accreditation, or regulatory agency of sentinel event
- ❑ Provide appreciation and recognition to solicited and non-solicited volunteers and to state and federal personnel sent to help

(Liaison Officer):

- ❑ Communicate final hospital status and termination of the incident to local EOC, area hospitals, and officials
- ❑ Assist with the repatriation of transferred patients

(PIO):

- ❑ Conduct final media briefing and assist with updating staff, patients, families, and others about the termination of the event

(Safety Officer):

- ❑ Ensure facility safety and restoration of normal operations

OPERATIONS SECTION

- ❑ Confirm water restoration plan with local water authority and complete microbiological testing and final potable water safety verification
- ❑ Restore normal patient care operations
- ❑ Ensure restoration of water and other infrastructure (e.g., HVAC)
- ❑ Repatriate evacuated patients
- ❑ Discontinue ambulance diversion and visitor limitations

PLANNING SECTION

- ❑ Finalize the Incident Action Plan and demobilization plan
- ❑ Compile a final report of the incident and hospital response and recovery operations
- ❑ Ensure appropriate archiving of incident documentation
- ❑ Conduct after-action reviews and debriefing
- ❑ Write after-action report and corrective action plan for approval by the Incident Commander, to include the following:
  - Summary of actions taken
  - Summary of the incident
  - Actions that went well
  - Areas for improvement
  - Recommendations for future response actions

LOGISTICS SECTION

- ❑ Perform evaluation and preventive maintenance on emergency generators and ensure their readiness
- ❑ Restock supplies, equipment, medications, food, and water
- ❑ Ensure that communications and IT/IS operations return to normal
- ❑ Conduct stress management and after-action debriefings/meetings, as necessary

FINANCE/ADMINISTRATION SECTION

- ❑ Compile a final report of response costs, expenditures, and lost revenue for approval by the Incident Commander
- ❑ Contact insurance carriers to assist in documentation of structural and infrastructure damage and initiate reimbursement and claims procedures

DOCUMENTS AND TOOLS

- ❑ Hospital Emergency Operations Plan
- ❑ Hospital Loss of Water Plan
- ❑ Hospital Loss of Sewer Plan
- ❑ Hospital Loss of HVAC Plan
- ❑ Facility and Departmental Business Continuity Plans

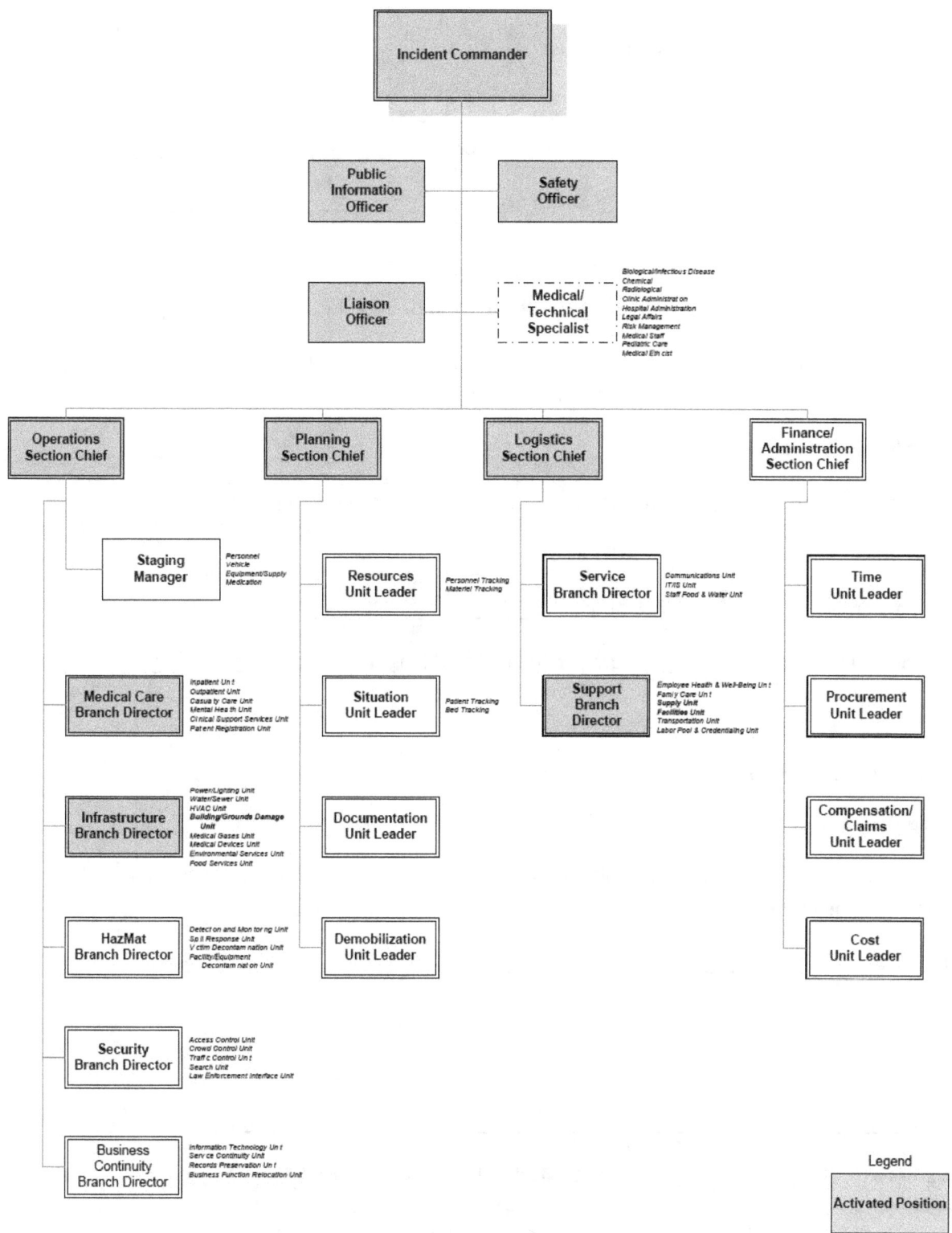

Figure C.1. Incident Management Team Chart (Immediate Operational Period 0-2 Hours)

Appendix D: Example Water Use Audit Forms 1 and 2

Department Water Use Audit Form 1 – Population

Date: _____Name(s) of staff completing form _____

Building #_____Dept. #_____ Level(s)/Wing(s) _____

Department Name/Function_____

Is there more than one major water-using activity in the department? (y/n)_____

If yes, how many?_____(Use additional pages to breakdown the population for each water-using activity and fill in the activity name/description below.)

Name/function of activity _____

Population: Departmental (only one activity/dept.) (y/n)_____or Activity (y/n) _____

(Enter the following data as DAILY AVERAGES)

Full-time employees _____8-hour shifts_____12-hour shifts_____

Part-time employees_____Average part-time shift length (hours) _____

Inpatients_____Occupancy Rate_____Visitors _____ Visitor stay (hours) _____

Outpatients_____Outpatient average stay (hours) _____

Can outpatients be temporarily postponed? _____ If yes, how many days? _____

Description of water-using activity: Explain critical water-using activities (i.e., water-requiring activity that cannot be interrupted).

Describe: _____

_____

Why is it considered critical? _____

_____

Water Fixtures Types: Faucets (F), Urinal (U), Toilet (T), Shower (S), Other (O)

Quantity of each: Faucets_____ Urinals_____Toilets_____Showers _____

Other _____

Other _____

Department Water Use Audit Form 2 – Activity Water Use

Date:_____Name(s) of staff completing form_____

Building #_____Dept. # _____ Level(s)/Wing(s) _____

Department Name/function_____

Activity Information: Department (only one activity/dept) (y/n)_____or Activity (y/n) _____

(Enter the following data as DAILY AVERAGES) (Use one form for each activity, if necessary)

Name/function of Activity_____

Description of activity: Explain critical aspects (must have water and not be interrupted).

Departmental (y/n) _____or Activity (y/n)_____

Describe: _____

_____

1. How much water used for each activity?   _____ units (e.g., volume per dialysis)_____

2a. Can water flow be measured/estimated? (y/n) _____ If yes, how long is the water used per activity? hrs._____ min._____

2b. How many times per day (D), week (W), or month (M)?   _____ per _____

3. Is this process essential for hospital operations (i.e., would loss of this function require partial or complete shut-down of the facility or the department)? (y/n)_____

4. Can the activity be temporarily postponed or substantially reduced in the event of a prolonged emergency? (y/n)___ If yes, how many days? _____

5. Are there waterless alternatives to the process? (y/n)_____ If yes, explain._____

6. Is the process dependent on water use in other hospital departments (e.g., operating room needs for sterile instruments)?_____

7. How long can the process operate without the need for outside water use (e.g., sterile instruments are in stock for how many procedures and/or days)? _____

8. When an emergency water shortage occurs in warm weather, is it possible to allow the air temperature to increase temporarily in the department without adversely affecting health or safety? (y/n) _____

9. Other comments:

_____

Appendix E: Portable Water Flow Meters

Where water usage information deficiencies are noted, either further personnel interviews or field observations will be required to asses water usage. As previously indicated, if the unaccounted for water exceeds 20%, the facility may decide to install portable flow meters to monitor water consumption in targeted buildings or areas. In situations where portable water meters are deemed necessary, the water use audit team may need to install transit-time flow meters at appropriate locations to measure and record flow within the pipe supplying the water to the targeted use(s). The use of temporarily installed water flow meters will assist in the determination of the unknown or difficult to estimate water demands.

The first step should be to conduct a tour of the facility to identify the number, locations, and logistical requirements for the installation of any temporary/portable flow meters that may be needed to obtain water usage information from specific areas within a facility. Examples of locations that might require the use of portable flow meters include:

- Power plant (This meter location can be the largest water use area at a health care facility.)
- Nephrology department (This meter location can be used to monitor dialysis water usage—in particular, the reverse osmosis [RO] system feed to the dialysis units. Data obtained can be used to determine/confirm average daily demand estimates for the dialysis high-purity water supply unit.)
- Service line(s) to operating rooms, including metering of water usage for instrument cleaning and sterilization equipment
- Representative outpatient departments (possibly two with the highest in-patient/employee count and an accessible and exclusive supply line)
- Representative inpatient departments (possibly two with the highest in-patient/employee count and an accessible and exclusive supply line)
- Restaurant/cafeteria (with all the associated water uses for food preparation, service, and cleaning)
- Psychiatric ward (for a representation of domestic water use in the ward)

The audit team, in coordination with the staff, should identify the final locations for portable flow meter installation based on water supply pipe layout and accessibility of a metering location directly upstream (if possible) of the water use to be monitored. The audit team will need to coordinate the final location(s) with the staff to ensure that pipes are properly prepared to facilitate meter installation and reading (e.g., insulation may have to be removed temporarily).

If temporary flow meters will be used, the appropriate instrumentation to be used during the water use audit should be obtained and calibrated. Note that the installation and calibration information provided with many of the temporary flow meters is not complete. To ensure that accurate information is obtained from these meters, it is recommended that the user contact the meter manufacturer for specific installation, calibration, and use instructions.

The installed and calibrated portable flow meter(s) can be used to record the water flow data for the targeted area. The audit team should plan to provide the maintenance staff with the final location(s) of the portable, transit-time flow meters at least one week before installation. The audit team will install the flow meters and ensure proper operation. The flow meters will continuously record potable water flow within the pipe for a period to be determined by the facility. Typically, the meters should be installed for at least one week. Extension of the flow monitoring period may be necessary, depending on the volume and quality of the flow meter data obtained.

www.ingramcontent.com/pod-product-compliance
Lightning Source LLC
Chambersburg PA
CBHW081830170526
45167CB00007B/2774